The Ultimate Prescription

Harnessing the Mind-Body Connection to Relieve Depression

ISBN: 1481865455
ISBN-13: 9781481865456
Library of Congress Control: 2012949226
Namaste Publications, Sacramento, CA

The Ultimate Prescription

Harnessing the Mind-Body Connection to Relieve Depression

John D. Winters &
Maxine Barish-Wreden MD, ABIHM
with Jason Warburg

Namaste Publications
2013

Dedication

To my grandfather and parents,
who inspired my journey

and

my wife Debra and our children Justin,
Ryan and Kayla, whom I constantly ask to discuss
our family goals and dreams.

—John D. Winters

To all people who have struggled to overcome
depression and anxiety.

—Dr. Maxine Barish-Wreden

TABLE OF CONTENTS

Foreword: Maxine Barish-Wreden, MD, ABIHM   ix

Introduction   xiii

Chapter 1: Everyone's Problem   1

Chapter 2: Unconventional Wisdom   9

Chapter 3: The Seven Hypotheses   17

Chapter 4: Breakthrough   23

Chapter 5: Sex & Chocolate   31

Chapter 6: Getting Started   39

Chapter 7: The Mind-Body Connection: The Power of Intention   45

Chapter 8: The Mind-Body Connection: Tools for Healing   55

Chapter 9: Your Food, Your Medicine   73

Chapter 10: Challenging the Paradigm   89

Chapter 11: The Revolution Starts Now   99

Chapter 12: The Ultimate Prescription   111

Afterword: John D. Winters   115

End Matter   121

Foreword

by Maxine Barish-Wreden, MD, ABIHM

I am passionate about the possibility of great health. As an internal medicine physician, I see dozens of people every week with chronic health problems that are largely brought on and influenced by the way we live our lives. Depression is no different, but many people think of depression as a genetic disease, something that can only be treated with drugs. This is far from the truth. I know, because I have struggled with my own mood swings for most of my life, and my own journey to find my way to contentment has led me to believe that depression is highly treatable without drugs. Many approaches can help to lift and keep people out of depression; exercise is one of those powerful approaches. The key message of this book is that most of you *can* help yourselves when it comes to battling depression, but it takes commitment and practice.

None of us would expect to earn a college degree without first committing to the course of study that it takes to earn that diploma. Yet when it comes to our own health, we often expect a miracle overnight when we start a new intervention or behavior, and we hope that once we start to feel better we will be able to return to our old ways of being, while still keeping the door prize. It's not just illogical, but crazy-making to think that we could do that. If you start to lift weights with the intention of lifting your mood or strengthening your muscles, and you go faithfully to the gym three times a week, chances are your biceps will respond beautifully to your workout, and you'll *feel* better–everywhere. If you slack off, however, you'll drop back to square one. Our minds and brains operate in much the same way—train your mind to think and process in a more uplifting and positive way, with practice and persistence you'll find your mood responding happily; stop your pursuits, however, and chances are you'll return to your pessimistic boot loop.

The good news: you *can* do just about anything you set your mind to. Okay, maybe you can't fly or grow a new arm. But really, most of us can create miracles in our lives. The bad news: yes, you have to work at it, you need to go for the gold, know what you want, declare it, claim your own healing–and then you need to take the required steps to turn things around for yourself. But hey, it's all about the journey anyway—there is no pot of gold at the end of the rainbow. There's only the satisfaction of knowing that you wrestled with something that was difficult for you, that you conquered your resignation and transformed your suffering into wisdom. And that, my friends, is the only thing we're really here for anyway.

We hope this book will open your eyes to some new and exciting research about exercise and depression, and also provide you with other useful tools for creating more satisfaction and joy in your life. The ball is in your court.

Introduction

You know someone who is depressed. You do. You might not even realize it, but you do.

It might be a friend tip-toeing through a crumbling marriage. It might be a co-worker feeling trapped by finances. It might be a family member whose chronic health problems have put them in a perpetual state of gloom.

It might be someone with no obvious challenges in their life, who is simply unable to pull themselves out of the quiet abyss of melancholy.

It might, for that matter, be the person reading these words, for reasons only you know, or maybe don't know, yet.

Whatever the case, you know someone who is depressed. And you want to help them. Of course you do. Anyone would.

We want to help you do that.

We have stood in your shoes (and you in ours). We come from families in which depression is as common as receding hairlines and terrible jump shots, self-deprecating humor and emotionally-charged family holidays.

And we could spend pages and pages here telling you about our own life experiences in excruciating detail—but that would be a different conversation and a different book. This book isn't about us; it's about you and how you can help that person you know, that person you care about, to feel better.

How can we be so sure that you know someone who's depressed? Because almost everyone knows someone who's depressed—it's one of the most widespread health problems in America today. We'll get to more facts and figures later on, but for now, consider just this one: more than one in 10 adults in the United States suffers from depression in any given year.[1]

Any problem affecting 10 percent of our population is by definition huge, and that's without even considering the spouses, family members, friends, co-workers and employers who are, effectively, collateral damage. As more and more people have come to recognize the scope of the problem, developing effective solutions to it has become both a pressing concern for doctors and big business for pharmaceutical manufacturers.

"Big business." Does that phrase leave you anticipating a rant against antidepressants? Sorry, but that's not what this book is about either. Antidepressants in and of themselves are neither good nor bad; they're simply a tool, and used judiciously under the supervision of a doctor, they can be quite beneficial. However, antidepressants also carry significant risks, including a variety of potential physical and mental side effects. Taking a wider view, they also carry substantial costs for patients, insurers, corporations and government health services.

The question this book asks—the question everyone should ask—is, what if there was a treatment for depression that didn't have those risks and costs associated with it, that anyone could give to themselves, that had only positive side effects, and that had been scientifically proven to be at least as effective in treating depression as prescription medications and conventional therapy?

Wouldn't you want to share the news about this "wonder drug" with a loved one suffering from depression—or use it yourself?

Wouldn't a treatment like that be the logical first step in addressing depression, before resorting to higher-cost, higher-risk alternatives?

And wouldn't that treatment be the sort of breakthrough that everyone who bears the costs of mental health care—from patients and insurers to corporations and the government—should get excited about?

Of course it would. But first, such a simple, low-risk, inexpensive treatment would have to exist.

The kicker is: it does.

☞☜

The treatment we're talking about is in fact so simple and logical and very nearly self-evident that when we mention it, people often smile and nod in agreement before we can even finish the sentence.

Exercise. The quote-unquote wonder treatment for depression is exercise.[2]

Of course, the very fact that it is so simple and logical and practically self-evident begs the question—if exercise truly is an effective treatment for depression, why aren't more mental health professionals prescribing it for their patients?

As is often the case with big-picture questions, here the past is as important as the present in shaping the future.

And so, in the early chapters of this book we'll walk you through the brief history of exercise as a treatment for depression, help you understand the science behind it, and explain the barriers that have until now prevented its acceptance by the medical establishment as a standard mode of treatment. Most importantly, we'll tell you about the recent study that fills in the blanks on the science of exercise and depression and conclusively proves how exercise affects the brain's mood center.

With that foundation established, we'll then walk you through some of the key hurdles depression sufferers face in employing exercise as a treatment, and recommend approaches for those ready to begin an exercise program.

Next, we'll examine the mind-body connection in greater detail and explore a broader range of natural remedies that can help alleviate depression, including meditation, journaling, experiencing nature and paying attention to nutrition.

Finally, we'll close with a few words aimed at the broader universe of professionals and policy-makers who have the power to reduce both the societal cost and the human cost of depression, if they'll simply adapt their thinking to the new science now in our hands.

We wrote this book with two goals in mind. First and foremost, we want to empower people suffering from depression, and their loved ones, with knowledge of the full range of proven treatment methods that are available to them. An empowered patient is an engaged patient and ultimately a healthier patient, and motivation and hope are two of the most important things you can offer to a person who is depressed.

A secondary goal is to sound the alarm to mental health practitioners, hospitals, insurance companies, employers and government policy-makers about the existence of a proven treatment method with the potential to revolutionize the way we treat depression. With the crisis in the American health care system worsening year after year, it's not just prudent but essential that we explore strategies that carry the potential to both help millions of people and save billions of dollars.

But before we get all wound up talking about societal costs and revolutionizing our health care system, let's remind ourselves: why is this so important? Why did we write these words, and why are you reading them?

Because, like us, you know someone who's depressed. You can sense their quiet suffering right now, this very minute, and more than anything, you just want to help.

Let's get started.

Key points of this chapter:

- **One in ten Americans suffers from depression.**

- Antidepressants are the tool many turn to first, but are just one of many tools available for treating depression.
- A remarkably effective natural remedy for depression exists: exercise.
- Our goal is to empower people suffering from depression (and their loved ones), with knowledge of the full range of proven treatment methods for depression.
- We also want to sound the alarm to mental health practitioners, hospitals, insurance companies, employers and government policy-makers about the existence of proven alternative treatment methods for one of the most prevalent and costly health problems in America today.

Chapter 1.
Everyone's Problem

The statistics on depression in America fall in the gap somewhere between stunning and jaw-dropping:

- More than one in 10 adults in the United States suffers from depression in any given year, and four out of five people suffering from mental disorders do not seek professional help.[3]

- Americans spend $13.5 billion annually on prescription antidepressants[4] and about $100 billion a year on psychological care.[5]

- In some states, the percentage of the population taking prescription antidepressants is as high as 14 to 16 percent,[6] despite the fact that up to 30 percent of depressed patients receive no relief from antidepressant medications.[7]

- The ripple effects of depression reverberate through the economy and society: in the health care system, depressed individuals typically spend 1.5 times more on health care costs than those who are not depressed;[8] in the workforce, researchers estimate that depression costs employers $44 billion annually in lost productivity.[9]

Things don't look much different across the Atlantic. In England, 25 percent of the population seeks medical care for mental health issues annually,[10] the National Health Service estimates the annual cost of mental health treatment at 32 billion pounds[11], and spending on prescription antidepressants rose over 2000 percent between 1993 and 2005.[12]

Now, consider the implications of these facts and figures when you start putting them together into a bigger picture.

Ten percent of the population means at least 30 million Americans suffer from depression—most of whom will never seek treatment for it. Meanwhile, most who do seek treatment are directed to take expensive and sometimes risky antidepressants. And all the while, both the treated and the untreated cost employers tens of billions of dollars a year in lost productivity.

Throw in spiraling healthcare costs, patchy coverage and an inadequate safety net and you have a genuine health care crisis, one in which patients grappling with depression may find it hard to get the help they need, and mental health professionals called upon to treat them may feel pressure to try for quick results with prescription medications rather than exploring alternative modes of treatment.

Once you consider not just the costs to the individual but the costs to society as a whole, the stark reality becomes clear: depression isn't just our problem, or your problem, or your friend's problem—it's everyone's problem.

৵৹

If depression is everyone's problem, then why isn't our health care establishment doing everything in its power to find better solutions to it?

They would likely be the first to insist that they are.

And when you asked them to expand on that, they would more than likely point to the same traditional therapies and medications we're all familiar with, as well as all of the research underway to try to build an even better antidepressant.

Chances are very good that exercise would not come up in the conversation at all.

Why is that?

To understand the reasons why our health care establishment has been and continues to be so resistant to the use of exercise as a treatment for depression, it's important to understand first just how much research has already been done on this topic, and what that research has found.

≈≈

When a health problem affects more than 10 percent of the population, you would expect a major research effort aimed at developing effective treatments for it.

That's true of depression, but not as true as you might hope. The situation is complicated by two factors.

First, a lot of people are squeamish about talking openly and honestly about mental illness. That complicates the researcher's task in every respect, from putting together a representative study sample to getting reliable information from the subjects involved.

Second, as a research topic, depression just isn't very glamorous. It's common, largely invisible and only occasionally and indirectly fatal. The nature of the beast is such that most of the time the medical establishment is only able to detect symptoms, not causes, and the small amount of basic physical evidence it's possible to collect about the condition comes from the very latest brain scans.

The biggest consequence of all these constraints is that much of the scientific research examining potential treatments for depression has been rooted in conventional wisdom and remained safely "inside the box." Most of the clinical studies on the books today have focused on variations on the same group of traditional treatment methods for depression, i.e. psychotherapy and psychiatric medications.

Now, as we said before, we're not opposed to using prescription meds to treat depression. To the contrary, we believe that both the scientific literature and years of practical application have proven that the right medications in the right dosage for the right patients with the right conditions can be a godsend. What we do believe is that, as a society, we have fallen hard for the idea of the quick fix, the "super-pill" that will instantly solve our problem, and that the medical establishment has not been immune to this trend. (For example, a study found the percentage of patient appointments psychiatrists devoted to psychotherapy fell from 44 percent in 1996-1997 to 29 percent in 2004-05.)[13]

Put another way, thinking outside the box doesn't always come easily for the medical establishment that by nature takes a conservative and very skeptical approach to new ideas.

Sometimes the box itself won't cooperate, though. Flaps pop open, sides collapse and new knowledge presents itself.

Such is the case with exercise. In course of decades of research examining various approaches to treating depression, an unexpected phenomenon gradually demanded the attention of more and more researchers—a phenomenon that many of the early trailblazers hadn't particularly intended to investigate, and that, even as more researchers began to focus on it, continued to defy scientific explanation.

What these doctors and scientists began to take note of in study after study was that one particular mode of treatment was surprisingly effective at combating depression—a treatment that was effective independent of either talk or drug therapy, and that carries none of the costs or risks associated with either one.

To return to the metaphor, you could say that when researchers were forced by the results in front of their eyes to start looking outside of the box, the first thing they saw was a shiny new pair of running shoes.

മ൭ഺ

Key points of this chapter:

- **Depression represents a huge cost burden on American society: $13.5 billion annually on prescription antidepressants, $100 billion a year on psychological care.**

- In some states, the percentage of the population taking prescription antidepressants is as high as 14 to 16 percent, despite the fact that up to 30 percent of depressed patients receive no relief from antidepressant medications.
- Depressed individuals typically spend 1.5 times more on health care costs than those who are not depressed; in the workforce, researchers estimate that depression costs employers $44 billion annually in lost productivity.
- The health care establishment continues to rely on antidepressants as the treatment of choice for depression despite increasing scientific evidence of the effectiveness of exercise as a treatment.

Chapter 2.
Unconventional Wisdom

The advice is as old as the hills: don't feel good? Take a walk and clear your head. (Maybe you even tried that one already.)

More recently, the media has talked up the "runner's high," which many athletes swear by, and almost as many scientists have dismissed as mythical.

And then there's the ultimate foundation underlying these almost instinctual approaches: humans were once hunter-gatherers whose very survival depended on staying active. From the dawn of our species, daily physical exertion has been hard-wired into our genetic code. Yet in the space of the last two or three generations, America has suddenly become a nation of couch potatoes, Internet addicts and armchair quarterbacks who view a trip to the grocery store as a major effort. At the same time, depression statistics keep rising, and might be rising even faster if more people sought help. Coincidence? We don't think so.

The first modern scientific study to look at the relationship between fitness and depression was a 1969 study in which Dr. W.P. Morgan noted a finding that feels somewhat obvious four decades later—as a group, depressed patients were less physically fit than the general population.[14] Norwegian researcher Egil G. Martinsen, one of the field's pioneers, picked up Morgan's thread a decade later and in 1979 confirmed his findings using a larger sample.[15]

The idea that there was some sort of inverse relationship between fitness and depression was in fact nothing new. Individual therapists as far back as 1905 had observed that exercise had positive effects on individual patients being treated for depression.[16] But it wasn't until Morgan and then Martinsen took up the chase that modern studies using statistically valid scientific methods began to take a closer look at the question.

A 1979 study by Morgan and a group of colleagues compared running with psychotherapy and found they were equally effective as treatments for depression.[17] A 1985 follow-up study established further that the patients who were enrolled in the initial study's exercise group "kept their gains better than those who attended psychotherapy."[18]

Several later studies produced similar results,[19] and before long a number of "meta-analyses"—scientific papers reviewing a collection of studies addressing a single subject—began weaving the various studies' findings into a set of informed conclusions. The meta-analysis produced by Gregg A. Tkachuk and Garry L. Martin of the University of Manitoba expresses the consensus conclusion as well as anyone's: "No controlled study has ever found exercise to be an ineffective primary or adjunctive treatment for mild to moderate depression."[20]

The next logical question was, how does exercise stack up against other treatment methods?

Martinsen noted that "later investigators have compared exercise to cognitive therapy and general counseling, finding them equally effective."[21] In 2000, Duke University researchers Michael Babyak and James Blumenthal divided a group of depressed patients into three: a group that took Zoloft, a group that took no medication, but exercised instead, and a group that did both. The results surprised even Babyak and Blumenthal: they found that a program of regular exercise was just as effective as medication in treating depression, and that patients who only exercised "were less likely to relapse than participants in the two groups receiving medication."[22] A more recent meta-analysis (2003) found that every relevant randomized study ever done demonstrated that exercise is in fact "equally or more effective than alternate interventions, including medication, psychotherapy, group therapy, or meditation/relaxation."[23]

Taking the comparative thrust even a step further, in 2004 Michigan State University researcher Lynette L. Craft achieved results similar to Babyak and Blumenthal's by adding regular exercise to the treatment regime of a sample group of women who had been taking antidepressants for an average of 47.3 months.[24]

Stop and think about that one for a minute.

The women in Craft's study had been clinically depressed for *years*. They had been using prescription medication as the primary treatment for their depression for an average of almost four years. They were still depressed—Craft describes their condition as "chronic depression." And yet they showed marked and lasting improvement within three weeks of starting an exercise program.[25]

Finally, Tkachuk and Martin deliver what ought to be the coup de grace in terms of earning the full attention of anyone who cares about both the human and the societal costs of depression: "Most notably, exercise therapy has proven to be four to five times more cost-effective than traditional treatments for depression."[26]

Let's review the math:

- One in ten Americans suffer from depression.
- Beyond that base, four in five people with mental health issues do not seek help.

- Americans spend more than $113 billion a year on therapy and antidepressants.
- Depressed people spend 50 percent more on health care than people who are not depressed.
- Exercise is four to five times more cost-effective than traditional treatments for depression.

If the problem is as widespread as the data suggest, the total economic impact of depression on American society could rival the annual federal budget deficit.

That doesn't change the fact that your primary worry when it comes to depression is your friend, or family member, or self. But considering the state of our economy today, it's mind-boggling to realize virtually no one in the public arena is demanding that we incorporate a proven, cost-effective remedy into standard treatment plans for a widespread condition that's a significant drag on worker productivity.

There are reasons for that. We mentioned two significant barriers before—the social stigma of mental health issues, and the lack of glamour (and grant funding) for researchers interested in studying non-pharmaceutical treatments for depression.

There is a third, and it's been a major roadblock ever since Morgan and Martinsen started looking at exercise as a possible treatment for depression.

The third major barrier is that, even with multiple scientific studies confirming that exercise is an effective treatment for depression, a fundamental question has dogged researchers from the very beginning. Science has proven beyond a shadow of a doubt that, as a remedy for depression, exercise works.

But *why* does it work?

స్త్రం

Key points of this chapter:
- **Human beings recognize on an instinctual level that movement and exercise makes us feel better.**
- **Scientific researchers have concluded in study after study since 1969 that exercise is an effective treatment for depression.**
- **Moreover, a number of studies have compared exercise to pharmaceutical approaches and found that exercise is as effective—often, more effective—than antidepressants for treating mild to moderate depression.**
- **There are three significant barriers to the adoption of exercise as a standard mode of treatment for depression:**
  - **Social stigma of mental health issues.**

o   **Lack of research funding for studies of exercise as a mode of treatment.**

o   **Lack of a scientific explanation of why exercise works.**

Chapter 3.
The Seven Hypotheses

The question of why exercise works as a remedy for depression is an absolutely vital piece of the puzzle here.

You don't want to just take somebody's word for something when it comes to your health any more than we or anyone else in our society wants to. Whether we're talking about physical health or mental health or both, we expect more. We want science—and its spokespeople, our doctors and mental health professionals—to tell us not just that the treatment they're recommending works, but how and why it works.

And that's where the catch-22 comes in as far as exercise and depression—when you have a treatment that you know is effective, but no one can explain why, people both inside and outside the medical establishment are going to be a lot more reluctant to recommend it.

The irony here is that we don't completely understand how many of the medicines that are typically prescribed to treat mental illness work. But because we've become conditioned in our society to taking pills and expecting results, we're perfectly willing to take a leap of faith and use prescription drugs to tinker with our brain chemistry, but the minute we hear about a therapist who installs a treadmill instead of a couch in her treatment room, we think they must be some kind of quack.

Most of the studies cited in our last chapter talk about different possible explanations for exercise being such an effective treatment for depression. There are seven main theories about why exercise helps, three that focus on psychological aspects and four that suggest physical or physiological origins:

- The Mastery Hypothesis
- The Distraction Hypothesis
- The Social Interaction Hypothesis
- The Fitness Hypothesis
- The Core Temperature Hypothesis
- The Amine Hypothesis
- The Endorphin Hypothesis

The Mastery Hypothesis is based on the idea that the act of mastering a skill—especially a skill the patient perceives as difficult—will reduce negative thoughts and trigger a more positive outlook. To be sure, depressed people who haven't been exercising regularly could experience psychological benefits from learning a new athletic skill and/or achieving the goal of exercising regularly. But the big flaw in this theory is that most of the studies that established the effectiveness of exercise as a treatment for depression involved routine, everyday forms of exercise such as walking and running. Most adults don't get a confidence boost from proving that they can put one foot in front of the other.

The Distraction Hypothesis could be summed up as "forget all your troubles" by doing things that you enjoy. The trouble with this theory is that research has shown that depressed patients experience greater improvement through a program of regular exercise than through self-identified "enjoyable activities."[27]

The Social Interaction Hypothesis suggests that engaging in a group activity and receiving positive reinforcement from peers could explain the positive effects of exercise on depression. Makes sense, right? Except that the data not only don't support it, they contradict it, finding that "subjects who exercised alone at home demonstrated larger decreases in depression than subjects exercising at other treatment locations (usually in groups)."[28]

The Fitness Hypothesis reaches back to the findings of the first Morgan study—that depressed patients were less fit than the general population—to try to find a direct relationship between depression and fitness levels. The data again don't support this, as the positive effects of exercise have repeatedly been found to appear within days, long before the subjects could have experienced any meaningful, lasting change in their fitness levels.[29]

The Core Temperature Hypothesis builds off of a couple of known facts: sustained exertion raises the body's core temperature by a degree or more, and increased core temperature tends to reduce muscle tension. Decreased muscle tension typically results in reduced stress and improved sleep patterns, which may help alleviate the symptoms of depression.[30] So: exercise equals core temperature rise equals decreased muscle tension equals relaxation equals reduced stress equals better sleep equals depression relief. Which is perfectly logical as far as Rube Goldberg chains of cause and effect go, but in reality is kind of like saying Henry Ford caused global climate change.

Of all the theories reviewed so far, the Amine Hypothesis might be the most intriguing one, and has been commented on favorably by both Morgan and Martinsen. Relatively recent discoveries about how the brain functions have revealed the key roles that three natural substances play in regulating mood and stress—serotonin, norepinephrine and dopamine. All three are what's known as monamine neurotransmitters, basically signal-callers in your brain's mood center. Most chemical antidepressants are believed to work by influencing the production and activity of these substances within the brain. And some studies on animals have shown that serotonin production increases during exercise.[31] However, there hasn't been enough research done in this area to come to any firm conclusions about how this theory might apply in the case of the positive effects of exercise on depression.[32]

To take it one step further, even if we assume that exercise triggers amine activity in the brain, the question remains—what's the mechanism? How does exercise change your brain chemistry?

Ah, but you've probably got another question on your mind right now: what about the Endorphin Hypothesis?

Key points in this chapter:

- **As a society, we have been more willing to take a leap of faith using antidepressants to tinker with brain chemistry than we have been to try alternative approaches that similarly lack a clear scientific explanation for how they work.**
- **Over the years, scientific researchers have put forth seven different hypotheses for why exercise is an effective treatment for depression.**
- **Six of the seven theories have significant flaws:**
  - o **The Mastery Hypothesis**

- o **The Distraction Hypothesis**
- o **The Social Interaction Hypothesis**
- o **The Fitness Hypothesis**
- o **The Core Temperature Hypothesis**
- o **The Amine Hypothesis**
- **The Endorphin Hypothesis has proven to be the breakthrough in understanding why exercise is an effective treatment for depression.**

Chapter 4.
Breakthrough

The term "endorphin" was coined in 1975 by Eric Simon as an abbreviation for "endogenous morphine," meaning "morphine produced naturally in the body."[33] Endorphins are opiates, as in opium, as in they are chemically similar to and related to morphine and heroin. The difference is, morphine and heroin are manufactured outside the body and then (usually) injected. Endorphins are produced inside the body and show up in both the bloodstream and the brain. They are quite literally a "natural high," your body's own organic mood enhancers.

From the time endorphins were first identified in the mid-1970s, they've been mentioned frequently in studies of the effects of exercise on depression. North, McCullagh and Tran cite a 1979 study by C.B. Pert and D.L. Bowie which found that exercise triggered a surge of endorphins. The surge was evidenced by "an increase in opiate (endorphin) receptor occupancy in the brain."[34] (Endorphin activity is typically measured by the availability of endorphin receptors in the brain—if they're available, there isn't much endorphin activity present; if they aren't, there's a lot of endorphin activity.) This might have been considered a breakthrough, if not for the fact that the subjects of Pert and Bowie's study were rats, and the endorphin activity in their brains was measured after they were dead.

The problem from the beginning has been that, throughout most of the period that researchers have been studying exercise a potential treatment for depression, the only way to measure endorphin activity in live human subjects has been in the bloodstream. In her excellent 2002 meta-analysis of exercise-depression literature, Amanda J. Daley cited Dr. Solomon Snyder's key 1977 endorphin study "The brain's own opiates," but noted that Snyder was only able to examine "peripheral endorphin levels (blood outside the blood-brain barrier) after exercise." Daley also cites a 1989 study which concluded that "because the blood-brain barrier blocks the passages by which 'opiate' substances move from the blood to the brain it is difficult to test the endorphin hypothesis."[35]

As if to illustrate the frustrations of researchers who knew they were onto something, but couldn't prove it yet, Michael Artal and Carl Sherman in 1998 argued in favor of using exercise as a treatment for depression, and pointed to the probable role of endorphins, while also lamenting that "[t]he ability of exercise to produce enough beta-endorphins to affect depression remains questionable."[36]

Artal and Sherman's frustrations also reflected the medical establishment's resistance to the new thinking represented by endorphin research. The more attention the media devoted to the endorphin surge generated by exercise—the "runner's high"—the more the medical establishment has resisted the practical implications of this phenomenon. In 1982, a Harvard physician went so far as to suggest in an article published by the *Journal of the American Medical Association* that the "runner's high" might be nothing more than a marketing ploy developed by sportswear manufacturers![37]

In spite of plentiful anecdotal evidence of the "runner's high" and consistent media interest in it,[38] researchers have continued to voice doubts about the endorphin hypothesis. As late as 2005, no less an authority than original "exercise as depression treatment" proponent E.G. Martinsen himself sounded unimpressed, saying that while exercise is associated with raised endorphin levels in the bloodstream, "[m]ost of the available experimental evidence in humans has not supported the endorphin hypothesis."[39]

So, as the calendar turned to 2008, the endorphin hypothesis remained just that—a theory, one of many. We knew that exercise elevated endorphin levels in the bloodstream, and we knew that exercise elevated the mood of the people doing it. But most researchers and medical professionals continued to resist the endorphin hypothesis because there was no concrete scientific proof that exercise triggers the release of endorphins inside the human brain.

There was no concrete scientific proof, that is, until now.

ॐॐ

Oddly enough, the breakthrough moment for the endorphin hypothesis didn't involve any of the major figures in exercise-depression research who we talked about in chapter two. Instead, it came from a group of German researchers who were curious about all the media coverage of the so-called "runner's high." If there was so much anecdotal evidence of this phenomenon, why hadn't anyone tested it properly to see if it really existed, and how it worked?

The roadblock—as we talked about before—had always been that researchers had no way of detecting the endorphin levels inside the brain of a living human being. (And we're pretty confident there were no volunteers to take the rats' place!) By 2008, though, a new method of measuring brain activity had come into play—positron emission tomography (PET) scans. PET scans are a safe, non-invasive way to track various biochemical changes in the brain. With their availability, researchers finally had the opportunity to measure endorphin activity in the brain, both before and after exercise, using live human subjects.

The German team, a group of nine researchers from the University of Bonn and Munich Technical University led by Henning Boecker, designed a very simple and straightforward experiment to test their hypothesis about the effect of exercise on endorphin activity inside the brain. Ten athletes were injected with the radioactive substance diprenorphine, which attempts to bind with the opiate receptors in the brain, basically competing for space with any endorphins present there. As Boecker explained it, "The more endorphins are produced in the athlete's brain, the more opiate receptors are blocked" from binding with the diprenorphine.[40] The PET scan is able to chart the location and volume of diprenorphine present in all areas of the brain.

Before and then again after taking a two-hour run, the ten test subjects each underwent a PET scan and filled out a questionnaire regarding their mood. In every case, the post-run PET scans showed "a significantly decreased binding" of the injected diprenorphine—in other words, exercise resulted in a significant increase in endorphins occupying and binding with the brain's opiate receptors, crowding out the diprenorphine.

And there it is—the missing piece of the scientific puzzle that has kept the medical establishment from accepting exercise as a scientifically supported treatment for depression. Exercise elevates mood by generating endorphins *inside* the human brain.

As important as this breakthrough was, it wasn't all the German research team found. The PET scans allowed them to see exactly which parts of the brain were being flooded with endorphins during and after exercise. Endorphin activity was concentrated in the prefrontal and limbic areas of the brain, which, as Dr. Boecker explains, "are known to play a key role in emotional processing."[41]

As if that wasn't enough to prove that exercise causes endorphin production causes improved mood, the results of the questionnaires filled out by the athletes before and after exercising seemed to clinch the argument: "[W]e observed a significant increase of the euphoria and happiness ratings compared to the ratings before the running exercise," noted Dr. Boecker. More importantly, his colleague Professor Thomas Tolle added that "the more intensively the high is experienced, the lower the binding of [the diprenorphine] was in the PET scan." In other words, "the ratings of euphoria and happiness correlated directly with the release of the endorphins."[42] The more endorphins are present, the more good feelings result.

The German team published the results of their groundbreaking experiment in the February 21, 2008 issue of the medical journal *Cerebral Cortex*, and on March 27, the *New York Times* published an article citing the study.[43] *Times* Reporter Gina Kolata sought comment from two American exercise researchers. One of the discoverers of endorphins, Johns Hopkins neuroscience professor Dr. Solomon Snyder, called the results "impressive." Huda Akil, a professor of neurosciences at the University of Michigan, summed up the outcome this way: "This is the first time someone took this head on. It wasn't that the idea was not the right idea. It was that the evidence was not there."[44]

But now it is. The supposedly mythological "runner's high" is no longer a myth, but a documented scientific fact.

We now know not only that the quote-unquote wonder treatment works, but how and why it works. The science is there. The only question left now is, what is it going to take to change the way we approach treating a condition that directly affects one in ten Americans, and indirectly affects the lives of millions more of us—family members, friends and co-workers?

Key points in this chapter:

- **Endorphins have long been considered a possible explanation for the positive effects of exercise on mood.**
- **However, scientists have lacked a method for measuring endorphins activity inside the living human brain.**
- **In 2008, a German study using positron emission tomography (PET) scans succeeded in measuring endorphin activity inside the brain before and after exercise.**

- **The study found a direct correlation between exercise and endorphin production, and endorphin production and elevated mood.**
- **Further, the study found that endorphins were present in the area of the brain most associated with emotional processing.**
- **The evidence is clear: the reason exercise counteracts depression is that it produces endorphins, which elevate mood.**

Chapter 5.
Sex And Chocolate

Now that we've explored the science of exercise and depression, we're left with—naturally—more questions. For example: it's clear now that exercise is an effective method of combating depression, and that endorphins are very likely the biological explanation for the way exercise elevates your mood. But is exercise actually the best and most practical source of endorphins for people who are depressed? If it is, why? And, how much is enough?

The answers are—maybe surprisingly, considering the subject matter—both interesting and more than a little amusing. And they start with another question.

Do you like chocolate?

Millions do. Millions of people swear it not only tastes good, it makes you feel good. It creates that proverbial warm fuzzy feeling inside, a genuine sense of contentment and happiness.

A sugar buzz, you might say? Not exactly.

While sugar probably plays a role, there's more to it than that. Because scientific research has shown that eating chocolate, besides delivering sugar and stimulating our senses of taste and smell, causes the human body to release endorphins.[45]

Yes, exercise does indeed have competition in the field of endorphin production! In fact, since endorphins were first discovered in 1975, science has proven that a number of fairly common activities beyond exercise and eating chocolate tend to trigger them.[46]

We know now that massage leads to increased endorphin levels.[47] Acupuncture—whose health benefits have been recognized for centuries, even if they've never been completely explained—has also been shown to be a source of endorphins.[48] And laughter gives endorphin production such a turbo-charge that even just the *anticipation* of laughter has been shown to boost endorphins in the bloodstream by 27 percent.[49] The old saying about laughter being the best medicine is truer than you might ever have imagined!

Assuming you took note of this chapter's title, though, you've probably been waiting for the final shoe to drop—presumably, on the bedroom floor. Alright, then; we won't keep you in suspense any longer. In a development that should come as no particular surprise to anyone, scientific researchers at Johns Hopkins University recently confirmed that endorphin production increases 200 percent during sexual activity.[50] Who says science is no fun?

҈

Of course, the reality that there are a variety of potential approaches to what some might call "endorphin therapy" does present some issues for those of us evaluating the mental health benefits of exercise.

The issue is basic. If endorphins really are the mechanism by which exercise improves mood, and if sex and chocolate also trigger the release of copious amounts of endorphins, who in the world is going to choose exercise from those three options? *"Let's see. I could head out the door at six a.m. for a three-mile run, or I could just climb back into bed with my lover and share a chocolate bar afterwards. Hmmm."*

That's where practical considerations come in. The downside of chocolate is clear—to generate the kind of mood-altering effects produced by exercise, you'd need to eat so much chocolate that your health would suffer in other ways. As for sex, like massage and acupuncture, it's an activity that's not necessarily available to everyone, and it's one that's even less likely to be available to a depressed person. (Not to mention the health risks involved in sexual activity outside a long-term monogamous relationship.)

Laughter and exercise, then, appear to be the safest and most universally available ways for a depressed person to generate endorphins. And while laughter is a wonderful thing and its health benefits should never be underestimated, it generally doesn't come easily for someone who is depressed.

Here we are again, then: back to exercise.

འ⊷ଋ

We don't want to make the case for exercise a negative one, though. In addition to being one of the most universally available sources of endorphins out there, it also has this big advantage: it only has positive side effects.

A brief digression on side effects here. You've probably been as amazed as we have by the sheer volume of commercials on television and the Internet over the last few years advertising prescription medications for depression and a hundred other ailments. The ads have become so common that as a viewer it's hard not to be skeptical about some of their claims, not to mention the sometimes exotic conditions they claim to remedy. The scary part, though, is when the narrator starts speed-reading down the list of potential side effects some of these medications carry—headache, nausea, joint pain, sudden drops in blood pressure and so on right up through risk of stroke, blindness, death and four-hour erections. At what point does the cure become worse than the problem?

Now imagine an ad script for the new treatment "exercise":

"Helps relieve depression. Side effects may include increased stamina and flexibility, improved muscle tone, reduced risk of heart disease, improved blood pressure, moderate weight loss, improved sleep patterns, enhanced libido."

Sounds like the proverbial wonder drug, doesn't it? As Dr. John J. Ratey puts it in his marvelous book *Spark: The Revolutionary New Science of Exercise and the Brain*, "If exercise came in pill form, it would be plastered across the front page, hailed as the blockbuster drug of the century."[51]

The one real risk associated with exercise is injury, and caution is definitely important when starting a new program of exercise, especially for someone who hasn't done it in a long time. So then, how much is enough?

A number of the same studies that helped to establish the benefits of exercise for mental health also measured the amount of time spent exercising that is required to achieve symptom relief. What's striking is how similar the results were in each case, and therefore how similar the resulting recommendations turn out to be. Psychiatrist Michael Artal recommends a goal of 20 to 60 minutes of walking or other aerobic exercise three to five times a week[52]. Drs. Andrea Dunn and Madhukar Trivedi advise "30 minutes of moderate intensity physical activity on most and preferably all days of the week."[53] The Mayo Clinic recommends "at least 30 minutes of exercise a day for at least three to five days a week to significantly improve depression symptoms."[54]

The irony is, these recommendations virtually duplicate the recommendations public health authorities worldwide have been making for years in an effort to foster optimum *physical* health. You could literally replace the word "physical" with "mental" in the typical public health recommendations and have them be just as accurate; in this case, what's good for the body is absolutely good for the mind as well.

That simple reality returns us to our hunter-gatherer ancestors and the question of whether human beings are defying thousands of years of biological adaptation when we choose not to be active. All the science we've reviewed so far in this book carries the same underlying theme—lack of exercise is a major cause today of not just physical but significant mental health issues as well. Most of the indicators point to the so-called "good life"–the laid-back, physically inactive lifestyle prevalent in modern Western civilization–as a sudden change in humans' habits that may literally be killing us. Human beings are meant to be physically active on a daily basis, and it's both unnatural and unhealthy for us not to be.

In the end, while there are many potential sources for mood-enhancing endorphins, and all are worth investigating, exercise offers the most complete package of low-risk, almost universally-available relief with only— and multiple—positive side effects. And those benefits are available with a commitment of just half an hour a day, several days a week.

The remaining question is obvious. If the benefits are clear and the time commitment required to achieve those benefits relatively small, why don't more patients—and the mental health professionals who treat them—take advantage of exercise as a baseline strategy for treating depression?

Key points in this chapter:

- **There are many ways to produce endorphins, but exercise is the most practical and easily available when compared to other options such as chocolate, sex, acupuncture, massage or laughter.**
- **Exercise also lacks any negative side effects; to the contrary, with the exception of the potential for injury, its side effects are all positive.**
- **The recommended amount of exercise to address depression symptoms—at**

least **30** minutes at least three times a week—mirrors the recommended guidelines for physical fitness.

- The only remaining question is, why don't more patients—and the mental health professionals who treat them—take advantage of exercise as a baseline strategy for treating depression?

Chapter 6.
Getting Started

Thanks to the Internet, we live in an era where so much raw information about medical conditions and modes of treatment and clinical studies is so widely available that it's not just possible but increasingly common for a highly motivated patient to be an active participant in their own diagnosis and treatment.

You're shaking your head already, though, and we know why.

For people coping with depression, one simple word in the above paragraph presents a huge roadblock—"motivated."

In the grips of depression, changing behavior becomes a much more difficult challenge than simply educating yourself and applying what you've learned. For people dealing with depression, the biggest hurdle is simply getting up off the couch.

The most important thing to understand for a depressed person who wants to try to help themselves is that you are not alone. Whether or not you have the benefit of a supportive counselor—and you should by all means seek one out—there are a number of excellent resources available for those ready to get up off the couch and get started trying to help themselves feel better.

In particular, the Mayo Clinic's Web site offers this framework for patients who want to incorporate exercise as part of their treatment for depression, available online at http://www.mayoclinic.com/health/depression-and-exercise/MH00043:

- **Get your mental health provider's support.** Some, but not all, mental health providers encourage exercise as a part of their treatment plan. Talk to your doctor or therapist for guidance and support. Discuss concerns about an exercise program and how it fits into your overall treatment plan.
- **Identify what you enjoy doing.** Figure out what type of exercise or activities you're most likely to do. And think about when and how you'd be most likely to follow through. For instance, would you be more likely to do some gardening in the evening or go for a jog in the pre-dawn hours? Go for a walk in the woods or play basketball with your children after school? Do what you enjoy to help you stick with it.
- **Set reasonable goals.** Your mission doesn't have to be walking for an hour five days a week. Think about what you may be able to do in reality. Twenty minutes? Ten minutes? Start there and build up. Tailor your

plan to your own needs and abilities rather than trying to meet idealistic guidelines that could just add to your pressure.

- **Don't think of exercise as a burden.** If exercise is just another "should" in your life that you don't think you're living up to, you'll associate it with failure. Rather, look at your exercise schedule the same way you look at your therapy sessions or antidepressant medication—as one of the tools to help you get better.

- **Address your barriers.** Figure out what's stopping you from exercising. If you feel intimidated by others or are self-conscious, for instance, you may want to exercise in the privacy of your own home. If you stick to goals better with a partner, find a friend to work out with. If you don't have extra money to spend on exercise gear, do something that's virtually cost-free—walk. If you think about what's stopping you from exercising, you can probably find an alternative solution.

- **Prepare for setbacks and obstacles.** Exercise isn't always easy or fun. And it's tempting to blame yourself for that. People with depression are especially likely to feel shame over perceived failures. Don't fall into that trap. Give yourself credit for every step in the right direction, no matter how small. If you skip exercise one day, that doesn't mean you're a failure and may as well quit entirely. Just try again the next day.

These guidelines are an excellent starting point for people who are ready to try the ultimate prescription for depression. We also strongly recommend Dr. Keith Johnsgard's *Conquering Depression & Anxiety Through Exercise* (Prometheus Books, 2004). Dr. Johnsgard, a retired clinical psychologist and professor emeritus at San Jose State University, illustrates of the effectiveness of exercise as a treatment for depression and related conditions, and in the last 20 pages of his book, offers specific suggestions for how to approach getting started with an exercise program.

Getting started will always be the number one hurdle for patients with depression. But for those who are able to take that first step, the process often becomes self-reinforcing:

"[D]epressed patients who are motivated enough to get help in many cases might be motivated enough to exercise on their own. And once they start, studies suggest many will get hooked. In surveys, people who exercise regularly cite as its main appeal its mental and emotional rewards. 'The most prevalent reason that people stick with exercise is its effect on mood,' says Andrea Dunn, a doctor of behavioral science whose research has focused on exercise."[55]

It's time to get started.

❧

Key points in this chapter:

- **The biggest roadblock to getting started on a course of treatment for depression that includes exercise is motivation.**
- **The Mayo Clinic's Web site offers an excellent set of guidelines for getting started, including finding a supportive mental health professional, setting reasonable goals, and being prepared for setbacks and obstacles.**
- **We also strongly recommend Dr. Keith Johnsgard's *Conquering Depression & Anxiety Through Exercise*, which offers specific suggestions for how to approach getting started with an exercise program.**

Chapter 7.
The Mind-Body Connection I: The Power Of Intention

You will succeed if you persevere, and you will find a joy in overcoming obstacles
- Helen Keller

While exercise is a vital component of well-being and a powerful tool in conquering depression, it is far from the only natural remedy available. The mind-body-spirit connection is another powerful tool we can engage in our quest for wellness. Neuroscientists are discovering that the brain, as well as the neuropeptides and neurotransmitters that are the language of the nervous system, are not fixed and static as we once believed, but are in fact fluid and malleable—capable of responding to the input they receive from our intentions, thoughts and actions. In the following two chapters, we'll review some of these new discoveries and introduce you to tools that, when practiced consistently, can create powerful changes in your brain and its chemistry, and ultimately in your mood and your well-being. You will come to see that you have far more power to create a life that you love than you may have ever given yourself credit for.

The vast majority of the research around mood and depression that has been done in the past 100 years or more has focused on depression and its treatment, especially with the use of medications; we have studied mental health in a pathological way, rather than thinking of mood as a human trait that exists along a spectrum. We have perpetuated the myth that some people are mentally ill, while others are normal, while in fact we all experience different levels of worry, anxiety, fear, and depression at different times of our lives. Many of us don't want to admit this, however, because of the stigma still associated with depression in our culture.

We have also thought of *good* mental health as simply the *absence* of depression. Until recently we have largely ignored the fact that we are indeed capable of cultivating much more positive mood states including happiness, contentment, and compassion. This ignorance has certainly been good news for pharmaceutical companies, who have profited from the sales of antidepressants, anxiety meds, and sleeping pills. It's bad news for you however, if you're one of the many people who have not responded to antidepressants, or have not had medical insurance to cover the cost of these meds, or who have had so many side effects from them that you have tossed in the towel and just decided to weather your mood storms without taking any drugs. And, recent research has suggested that for mild to moderate depression, anti-depressants are in fact no more effective than a placebo pill[56].

Another thing that kept us stuck in the medical-pharmaceutical model of treating depression was the belief that the brain was pretty much a fixed and unchangeable structure after childhood. If you happened to have been cursed with bad genes, bad exposures, or bad luck, then once your brain growth was complete you were stuck with that brain for the rest of your life. In the later part of the last century however, scientists began to discover that the brain in fact is malleable and changeable. Up until that point, it was believed that the wiring of the brain stopped around the age of 3, and that a child's brain reached full maturity around the age of 12. Scientists then discovered that a child's brain actually kept growing and maturing into the mid 20s, especially in areas of emotional growth, impulse control, etc. Surely though, the brain was fixed after that, right? Turns out the answer is no—far from it, in fact.

In the 1990s, an explosion of neuroscience studies turned our ideas upside down. We discovered two major important facts about the brain. First, the brain is in fact never fixed, but can change and grow throughout our lifetime; this concept is called neuroplasticity. In other words, the brain is a soft plastic organ that can be molded or shaped depending on the input provided to it; it is also capable of overcoming damage inflicted upon it. For example, if a particular area of the brain is destroyed by a stroke, say the area that controls language, scientists have discovered that with devoted attention and intention, other parts of the brain may be recruited to learn the damaged area's function. We can regain skills that we may have lost.

The other major concept that has shaken up our beliefs about the brain is called neurogenesis. Neurogenesis means that the brain can actually give birth to completely new cells, that it can grow and recruit new cells to replace ones that have died from old age or from damage to the brain. Initially it was felt that only certain areas of the brain could do this, but newer research suggests that multiple areas of the brain are capable of creating new cells. Research has also shown that suppression of neurogenesis can lead to mood disorders including depression and anxiety. Many things can suppress neurogenesis, including early life or prenatal stressors, inflammation, or chronic illnesses such as diabetes, hypothyroidism, sleep deprivation, excessive alcohol consumption, and stress. What helps to promote neurogenesis? Exercise, as you may have guessed, is a potent stimulator. Reducing chronic stress and illness, and staying actively engaged in life, are also useful. Prescription anti-depressants also seem to exert their benefit at least in part through neurogenesis[57].

So, now that we've seen that the brain has the capacity to grow and change throughout our lifetime how do we make practical use of these discoveries in our own lives, especially when we've been plagued by our swinging moods? Some of the answers to these questions may be found in the ancient teachings of the meditation traditions of the east.

Primarily based on a series of meetings and scientific investigations between neuroscientists, the Dalai Lama, and monks who have meditated for thousands of hours, we have discovered that the brain responds to our intention to be well, to be content and happy, and to compassion. And, the more we practice and cultivate these nourishing mind states, the more the brain physically changes and the more our brain communication chemicals, or neurotransmitters, change[58].

Three areas in the brain are apparently of crucial importance in this dance. The left prefrontal cortex (just behind the left forehead) seems to be the area of the brain tuned to happiness, while the amygdyla (in the deep middle part of the brain) is the center of emotion and stores negative emotions. The hippocampus is one area of the brain where new cells are formed (neurogenesis) and may serve as a way station between the other two. When we are chronically stressed or depressed, the hippocampus shrinks and cannot make new brain cells very efficiently. The prefrontal cortex also shrinks while the amygdyla tends to enlarge. Conversely, the hippocampus expands in response to meditation and compassion.

So what does this mean for those of us who have struggled with depression? Well, there's good news as well as bad news here. The good news is that we probably have far more of an impact on our moods than we may previously have given ourselves credit for. The bad news is that we may truly be responsible for our well being—i.e., if we want to get better and stay well, it will mean choosing to be well and committing to the path and practice of mind-body techniques that will help to modulate our moods.

The field of psychology has really shifted in the past 20 years or so alongside these discoveries; whereas we used to talk about "toxic parents" and other tales of woe that we were sure explained our neuroses and unhappiness, psychology has now finally entered the happiness field. And, the discoveries parallel those of the brain scientists—when we put our attention on the good in our lives, on our strengths, on joy and laughter, we not only cultivate those traits in our lives, we also change the circuitry, anatomy, and chemistry of the brain—we begin to see the power that we have to create what we want for ourselves. But this takes intentionality, practice, and persistence–we must keep our eyes on the prize while we cultivate tools of peace, contentment, and patience on a daily basis.

In this and the following chapter we'll review some of these practices that have been shown to be powerful antidotes to depression and anxiety. We'll also review some highly recommended books, CDs, and programs that can be wonderful guides to you on this journey, especially when the path does not seem well lit.

So let's begin with intention.

Intention

When we are ill, when we are out of sorts, or when we are depressed, when we find ourselves out to sea and rudderless, it can feel impossible to see where we'd like to go, to see a destination. However, without a firm intention to get well, we are more likely to flounder or to suffer for a longer period of time.

Getting well again almost always necessitates a declaration, a strong intention to heal, a pronouncement of a new path, even if one cannot see it. Many people who have recovered against all odds can attest to this. Sometimes, we start when a good friend refuses to see us stay defeated; sometimes some serendipitous event occurs and we are able to hear a call to action or to opening that had long been muffled. Sometimes it means surrendering to our true selves and letting go of ways of being, habits of lifestyle, or paths of action that no longer serve us and no longer authentically express who we really are (*your truth* will set you free). Sometimes it is an act of faith, or we hear it as the voice of our heart or our guide or our God, calling to us, calling us back home to our worthiness and our magnificence and our power. Sometimes it may feel like an act of Grace.

But no matter how it shows up for you, the key idea here is to get crystal clear on your intention right from the start, because without getting clear on our intentions, we tend to flounder, to stay on the fence, and to avoid the committed actions that will lead to the outcome we desire. In fact, If you find yourself stuck and unable to move forward, you might get some insight by making a list of the benefits you accrue for yourself by staying stuck—e.g., what's the payoff to staying depressed? Do you get to hide out? Avoid responsibility in your life? Avoid taking risks or going after dreams?

The quotes below sum this up nicely:

Until one is committed, there is hesitancy, the chance to draw back, always ineffectiveness. Concerning all acts of initiative (and creation), there is one elementary truth the ignorance of which kills countless ideas and splendid plans: that the moment one definitely commits oneself, the providence moves too. A whole stream of events issues from the decision, raising in one's favor all manner of unforeseen incidents, meetings and material assistance, which no man could have dreamt would have come his way.
—W. H. Murray in *The Scottish Himalaya Expedition*, 1951

Whatever you can do or dream you can, begin it.
Boldness has genius, power and magic in it!
—Johann Wolfgang von Goethe

So, what can you boldly declare for yourself right now about your intended future? You may want to make a list of what you want for yourself, or of where you intend for your life to be a year from now. If you find yourself stuck, think about what you dreamed of doing or being when you were a young child—in our younger years, we're usually unencumbered by self-doubt, and are more likely to authentically express what we're here to do on this earth. If that doesn't help, then make a "bucket list"—a list of things that you want to do before you die—and start with one of the things on your list. To further the action on this, make a collage of what you intend for your life to look like in 6-12 months; what actions will you have taken, where will you be living, how will you look, etc.

Once you've established clear intention and commitment to this path, you're ready to take the next steps toward healing.

ॐॐ

Key points in this chapter:

- **Research about and treatment of depression has been held back for years by the stigma associated with mental health issues and gaps in understanding regarding moods and brain chemistry.**
- **Mood exists along a spectrum, and it is possible to cultivate a positive mood state without chemical assistance.**

- **The brain is not a fixed structure, but can change and grow throughout our lifetime.**
- **The more we practice and cultivate positive mind states, the more the brain and its neurotransmitters physically change.**
- **We probably have far more of an impact on our moods than we may previously have given ourselves credit for—however, this also means that if we want to be and stay well, we must choose and commit to practices that promote positive mood states.**
- **The first necessary step is intention, a commitment to follow through and take a leadership role in your own healing process.**

Chapter 8.
The Mind-Body Connection II: Tools for Healing

Now that you've gotten your intention clear, let's explore a range of additional mind-body tools to see which, if any, might be useful for you in this healing journey.

Meditation

Have you ever heard the term "neurons that fire together, wire together"? It is sometimes called Hebb's rule, after Donald Hebb, PhD, the psychologist and neuroscientist who showed that neurons connect together more efficiently when they repeatedly fire together. In other words, when nerves are stimulated over and over down a certain path, they tend to cluster together in networks of nerves that then become activated easily. What does this mean for someone who is depressed? It means that one stressful thought can lead to your brain cascading down a river of self-doubt that magnifies that thought, pulling you down into another episode of depression. Byron Katie, the well-known spiritual teacher, describes this as "the thought that kicks you out of heaven." Most of us who've ever been depressed can relate to this.

But, before you let that thought take you down the depression trail again, consider this: meditation training can help you to alter those boot loops in a couple of ways. First and foremost, meditation trains you to observe your thoughts without getting caught up in them, believing them, or assigning them any meaning. Meditation training provides other benefits as well. If the intent of your meditation practice is concentration, you will become more focused in your day; if your intention is peace, you will generate more calmness in your life. And if your focus is on the compassionate relief of suffering in the people around you, you will feel more connected to others, and you might even find yourself more engaged in altruistic behavior such as volunteer work. The key here is intention, cultivation, and practice. In order for us to change the connections in the neurons in our brain, and to strengthen the connections that create peace and joy in our lives, we must practice this on a daily basis. The good news is that practice and cultivation lead to changes in our wiring, changes in the brain's tissue itself, and ultimately lasting changes in our experience of well-being and happiness.

The other powerful thing about meditation is that it allows us to see the transient nature of events in our lives and in our minds. When you become the observer of the thoughts that pass through your consciousness, you notice that everything is continually changing—

thoughts, emotions, bodily sensations—everything continually in flux and motion; nothing lasts forever. You also come to see that suffering arises mainly when we get grasp and try to hold on to something—for example, you latch on to a painful thought and hold onto it like a hot coal, rather than observing it and letting it pass. Or you might get attached to a good feeling or to a relationship and not want to let it go. We let go of suffering when we let go of our attachment to things and learn to trust more in the flow of life just as it shows up. We can learn to ride the tiger so to speak, without getting trampled in the jungle of our thoughts[59].

Prayer

Prayer can also be a powerful way to generate feelings of well-being, peace, and gratitude. For some people, a prayer is like a simple meditation—a focus on a particular word or phrase, and a return to that phrase when the mind wanders—e.g., using rosary beads helps to keep the mind focused while in prayer. Another powerful way of using prayer during times of depression is to ask God for insight or guidance, for acceptance, and for peace. This helps us to cultivate the idea that all things happen for a reason, that every challenge in our lives has a hidden gift for us, and if we can learn to stay present with how things are and to trust that good will emerge, we will be graced with expansion and with a renewed sense of ourselves.

Gratitude

Let's explore another simple practice that has the power to blow away the blues. That practice is

Gratitude. Gratitude has long been considered an integral part of a spiritual and a whole life in many traditions and cultures, but scientists have only recently studied the impact of a gratitude practice on one's well-being or measure of happiness.

Some of you may remember the "Toxic Parents" approach to psychology that was popular in the 1980s—identify what was toxic in your upbringing so you could blame your parents for all of the woes in your life. The problem with this approach was you might have felt a little better in the short-run by having a good rant about your parents, but chances are your feelings of shame, depression, or inadequacy would soon rear their heads again. Why is this? It probably harkens back to the concept mentioned earlier in this chapter about neurons firing and wiring together. When we focus on what we don't want or don't like about ourselves, our families, and our lives, we tend to generate and strengthen those emotions and outcomes, and we often miss all of the abundance and gifts that lie right before us and around us. We also develop tunnel vision about the people in our lives, so that all we may see are their faults; they have no room to offer us love, and if they did, we would surely reject is—this allows us to keep our dramas and stories running. Again, this may feel good, or even justified, in the short run, but in the long run we are only harming ourselves—we are cutting ourselves off from others in the world, and at the same time we continue to wound *ourselves* by failing to accept and love the parts of us that can also be hurtful and unkind. And—just so you don't take your negative thinking too personally, consider that some scientists believe that we actually enter this human existence already hard-wired for criticism and pessimism—after all, primitive people who were always on the lookout for danger probably had a survival advantage. We cannot rid ourselves of judgment and criticism, but we can learn to observe these thoughts and emotions, to see where they might occasionally provide us with useful information, and to balance them with acceptance and equanimity.

So where does gratitude fit in here? Gratitude is the antidote and the balancing potion for the pessimistic pathways in our brain. The practice of gratitude shifts the lens through which we view life from scarcity, anger, and fear towards abundance, appreciation, and awe. When we focus on gratitude, when we stop and deliberately name all of the things that we are grateful for during the day, we start to see instead all of the good in our lives, to see that the good in reality far outweighs any of the negative.

So what's the bottom line? Gratitude researchers, including folks like Robert Emmons, PhD, at the University of California Davis, have shown that the practice of gratitude has a profound impact in our lives. They have found that people who cultivate a gratitude practice in their lives have:

- More friends and stronger social support networks

- More satisfying and longer marriages
- Less stress, isolation, and loneliness
- More energy, better quality sleep, and better physical health
- More work productivity and better quality work
- Improved academic performance
- Greater longevity

People who practice gratitude even exercise more and have better athletic performance. What a simple, profound, and inexpensive way to boost your mood and enhance your well-being! A simple way to begin cultivating gratitude in your life is to make a list at the end of your day of everything you were grateful for about that day; include in particular the small things that you noticed—the smile you received from your child, your first cup of coffee or tea in the morning, the gentle touch of a friend, etc.[60]

In ordinary life we hardly realize that we receive a great deal more than we give, and that it is only with gratitude that life becomes rich.—Dietrich Bonhoeffer

To see an extraordinary video on gratitude, go to http://www.gratefulness.org/brotherdavid/a-good-day.htm

Forgiveness
Of the seven deadly sins, anger is possibly the most fun. To lick your wounds, to smack your lips over griev-

ances long past, to roll over your tongue the prospect of bitter confrontations still to come, to savor to the last toothsome morsel both the pain you are given and the pain you are giving back—in many ways it is a feast fit for a king. The chief drawback is what you are wolfing down is yourself. The skeleton at the feast is you.

—Frederick Boehner

When I have forgiven myself and remembered who I am,
   I will bless everyone and everything I see
   - A Course in Miracles

Every one of us has experienced hurt in our lives; perhaps we were abused in some way as children or as adults; perhaps we have felt betrayed, rejected, or humiliated by a family member, friend, or boss. No matter what the source or reason for our hurt, holding onto our grudges and grievances eventually hurts only one person: ourselves.

There is now a growing body of scientific evidence about the power of forgiveness to help us heal, both emotionally and physically. Conversely, there is evidence that anger, resentment, and hostility can adversely affect our health; unresolved anger and grievances can increase our risk of heart disease, high blood pressure, infections including colds, fatigue, headaches, and arthritis pain.

So, how do we begin the process of forgiveness? Many people are reluctant to forgive because they believe that forgiveness implies reconciliation with the one who hurt you, or condoning a harmful act that was perpetrated. However, forgiveness begins with the *willingness* to surrender our resentment, to let go of how we thought life *should* have been, to examine our stories more objectively.

Dr. Fred Luskin, Ph.D., director and co-founder of the Stanford University Forgiveness Project, defines forgiveness as "the feeling of peace that emerges as you:
- Take a hurt less personally
- Take responsibility for how you feel
- Become a hero instead of a victim in the story you tell."

Forgiveness begins to emerge when we recognize the human-ness of the people around us, including ourselves:
- No one is perfect
- We all make mistakes
- We have all done things to harm ourselves and harm others in the past
- None of us is alone in this regard.

When we can embrace this, we can begin to develop a sense of compassion for ourselves and the world, we can begin to re-invent ourselves, to become the hero of our own stories, instead of being stuck in our past hurts.

For an added bonus, consider what role you may have played in any relationship from the past that still stings; the person you need to forgive the most may be yourself. When you are ready, you might even want to speak with or meet with that person if possible to put things to rest. If that person is no longer alive, then writing a letter is sometimes a good substitute[61].

Guided imagery

The human imagination can be a powerful healing tool. We often think in images, and those images can evoke powerful emotions that lead to changes in our bodies. Just think about what happens in your body when you imagine sucking on a lemon—most of us will experience physical changes in the mouth from this image. Your lips may pucker, your face may contort, and your salivary glands go into high gear—and all because of the rich imagery and associations in your mind from your past experience with a lemon. Painful emotions and images from the past also affect us physically—when we conjure up those memories, we may find ourselves right back in the painful moment as if it were happening again right now—we can end up anxious, depressed, and in more physical pain. Guided imagery is a healing technique that helps to deliberately create positive, healing images to counteract these negative ones. During guided imagery, you listen to either a recorded or a live voice of a guide or therapist who first helps you achieve a state of deep relaxation. Once you are relaxed, your guide will help you to travel into the part of your body or psyche/soul that is in pain, and ask it what it needs from you—here you are engaging your deep inner wisdom or intuition to help you to heal. You may also use imagery to direct your own inner healing resources to that part of your body-mind or your life that you would like to transform.

Studies have shown that guided imagery can help to reduce pain, anxiety, and depression. It has also been shown to lower blood pressure, help people to heal more quickly from surgery, lose weight and quit smoking[62]. (6)

For more information, or to find a qualified guided imagery therapist, go to

http://www.academyforguidedimagery.com/index.html

http://belleruthnaparstek.com/

Journaling

Some experts say that depression is anger turned inward on ourselves. Many of us have a hard time accepting our dark emotions—anger, jealousy, greed, etc.—and if we don't find safe ways to accept and work with strong feelings like these, we may turn them inward on ourselves—kind of like our own inner torture chamber. One way through this is to journal your thoughts and feelings, especially with the intention of releasing them and clearing them from your body-mind. This is usually referred to as "expressive writing." On paper, you can write out every nasty, mean, or uncomfortable thought or feeling you've ever had, and get it out of your psyche.

When you're done, you can even create a ritual of release by burning or shredding what you've written—it was only meant for your eyes anyway.

Dr. James Pennebaker at the University of Texas has been one of the world's leading researchers in the positive impact of journaling on healing. He and others in the field have found that expressive writing can reduce physical symptoms and help people to get better from numerous conditions, including depression, asthma, rheumatoid arthritis, immune dysfunction, and HIV infection[63]. His book *Writing to Heal* is an excellent beginning guide for anyone interested in the benefits of this kind of work[64].

Nature

Studies have shown that being outside in nature can also improve your mood, and if you throw some exercise in as well, you'll get even more benefit. Scientists at the University of Essex found that people were less angry, depressed, and stressed after exercising outside; their self-esteem improved as well. Exercising near a body of water seemed to enhance the benefits of nature even more[65]. All of these benefits are in addition to what one would normally get by exercising inside. How easy can it get?

Sleep

Restful sleep is very important in the treatment of depression and anxiety. Getting a good night's rest will enhance your mood and well-being, while chronic sleep deprivation increases your risk of anxiety and other mood disorders[66]. For some people, sleep deprivation occurs because we over-schedule ourselves, and just don't make the time for adequate sleep and rest. For many others however, insomnia has become a chronic problem—it may be caused by anxiety or depression, it may be due to a primary sleep disorder such as restless leg syndrome, or it may be caused by other medical problems including sleep apnea, heart disease and arthritis. It's important to speak with your physician and to get treatment for insomnia. You may need a sleep study to rule out a primary sleep disorder, you may need treatment for any contributing medical conditions, or you may simply need some structure and coaching in creating a more healthy sleep pattern.

Pet therapy

We're sure that many of you are not surprised by the fact that pets can help to reduce anxiety and depression. In fact, many hospitals have pet therapy programs, known as "animal-assisted therapy," to help reduce the stress and anxiety that are associated with being in the hospital. Guide dogs are even being used now to help people with post-traumatic stress disorder[67]. If you are an animal lover and you suffer from depression, keeping a pet is an idea worth considering.

Laughter and Play

Laughter—the best medicine! Cultures from the ancient Greeks to Native Americans have long recognized the power of humor to help us to heal. Studies of laughter have shown that laughter, both spontaneous and planned, has multiple health benefits, including reducing our stress hormones, increasing our endorphins (nature's own natural pain-killers), reducing physical and mental pain[68], and increasing our sense of optimism. Laughter also helps us to take our lives a little less seriously, and when we do that, we open up space for creative problem-solving so that we don't stay stuck in whatever funk we may find ourselves. Laughter and play also stimulate the vagus nerve, which leads to the secretion of oxytocin from the pituitary gland, and oxytocin is the hormone of human bonding—it enhances connectivity between people, especially between mothers and their babies. It also increases one's sense of trust in others.

What should you do if you want to become more mirthful or playful? Don't worry—you don't have to become a stand-up comic! In fact, people who learn to find and appreciate the humor all around them seem to benefit the most (that's right—humor is a *learned* behavior—you too can do this!). Start by learning to take yourself less seriously and hanging out with people who make you laugh. Spend time with a five-year-old and rediscover the playful aspects of everyday life. You can even take on a daily laugh-practice: laugh from your gut for 30 seconds without stopping; when you master that, go for a full minute or more; you'll find that it's hard to stop once you really get going. In fact, Dr. Madan Kataria in India created "Laughter Yoga" in the 1990s as a means of helping his patients to reduce stress and anxiety and to heal. There are now Laughter Yoga clubs all over the world where people gather for 30-60 minutes of therapeutic laughter a day; perhaps joining one of these clubs is just the mood cure for you (http://www.laughteryoga.org/).

Massage Therapy

Massage therapy has also been shown to reduce depression, and oxytocin may be the key here as well. Anyone who has had a therapeutic massage knows how good it feels to be lovingly touched by another human being. It turns out that compassionate human touch, like laughter, also enhances the secretion of oxytocin, which is probably why massage enhances mood[69]. And when you consider that the cost of a one-month supply of antidepressant medications will pay for at least a few massages, then touch therapy seems like a bargain treatment for depression!

Singing

Studies suggest that both singing as well as listening to music can enhance mood. Ever been to a gospel music festival? We have noticed that it is almost impossible to feel depressed when you are in the midst of powerful music, especially music that you love. The benefits of singing are similar to those of laughter—improved mood, reduced stress, and enhancement of our immune system[70].

Community and connectedness

Staying connected with your family, friends, and work or social groups is a powerful antidote to depression and loneliness. We are creatures of community, and we are also here to share our gifts and talents with the world, and when we don't do this we can easily get depressed. That's one of the reasons why volunteer work helps to heal depression—it allows us to contribute to others, and it also helps us to take the focus off of our own suffering. In fact, the famed psychiatrist Carl Menninger reportedly said that he could cure anyone of depression in two weeks, simply by taking that person to the poorest part of town and having them do volunteer work with people who were less fortunate.

Reframing: Shifting from being the victim of your circumstances to becoming the hero of your own life's journey

Finding a new way of viewing an old problem in your life can be profoundly healing. This has been called reframing–putting a new frame of mind or a new spin on an old, persistent, or painful story. Here's one way to put this into action: imagine yourself sitting in the theatre of your life as an audience member, and witnessing the story of your life on stage, with you as the central character, the hero of your own journey. Imagine that you are also the director of this drama, as well as the casting director. You have written the story, cast all of the characters, and designed the sets, the scenery, and the costumes. You have ensured that your hero will have the perfect mix of adventure and pleasure, pain and challenge. With a bird's eye perspective, be a compassionate witness to your own life—what strengths have you given your character? What flaws? What profound lessons will he or she have to grapple with? How will these lead to insight and growth? If you don't like how the story is unfolding, consider that you can rewrite the script. You can also rewrite your interpretation of the events, and re-cast them as necessary to the spiritual growth and evolution of your character. Sometimes just shifting the perspective of your life in this way can be profoundly healing.

Becoming Your Own Best Friend

The pain of depression can make it hard to see any goodness in ourselves. But it helps to remember that self-condemnation is just a story that we get sucked into when we're feeling down, and it's never the truth. To paraphrase the renowned meditation teacher Jon Kabat-Zinn, "The fact that you are here, now, means that there is far more that is working well in your life, far more that is good about you *now*, than not good". Recovering from depression is enhanced when we take *responsibility* for acknowledging that good, and for acknowledging the gifts and the contributions that we make in the world. And ultimately, healing also means that we compassionately acknowledge and embrace those parts of ourselves that are less skillful and less acceptable, because they are also a part of our wholeness, and of our richness. When we befriend the full spectrum of who we are with kindness and compassion, when we say "This is who I am, *and it's ok*", when we share our gifts with the world, and allow the world to share its abundance with us, then we will truly be healed.

We hope that some of these tools will be useful for you on your journey. We know that with intention, practice, cultivation, and action, you can create miracles in your life.

౼৵

Key points in this chapter:

- **The mind-body connection offers numerous useful tools for treating depression. They include:**
    - o **Meditation can help you concentrate, focus and let go of negative emotions.**
    - o **Practices such as prayer and gratitude can help us focus on positive aspects of our lives.**
    - o **Guided imagery and journaling may help us identify and release negative emotions and experiences.**
    - o **Addressing environmental influences through experiencing nature, allowing for human touch, fostering better sleep patterns and/or pet therapy may improve mood.**
    - o **Activities such as singing, laughter and connecting with one's**

        community can generate a more positive frame of mind.

    o   **Reframing life events in a more positive way can help you to shift from being a victim to being the hero of your own story.**

- **You can use these and other tools to take charge of your own life's journey and shift the perspective of your life.**

Chapter 9.
Your Food, Your Medicine

Let food be your medicine and medicine be your food. Nature heals; the physician is only nature's assistant.

—Hippocrates

Exercise and body-mind-spirit interventions are powerful tools when it comes to preventing and treating depression. But food and supplements also have a significant impact on mood. In this chapter, we'll go over some key ingredients to keep your body-mind in tip-top shape.

A Whole Foods Approach

If you take a look around your average grocery store these days, you'll see thousands of processed products on the shelves. Many of these foods, if we can even call them foods, contain a list of chemical ingredients that your great grandmother wouldn't even recognize as edible. This massive change in the processing and marketing of food has taken place in a relatively short period of time compared with how humans have eaten since the beginning of civilization. Since the mechanization of agriculture and the USDA support of the massive production of corn and soy in particular, our food markets have been glutted with cheap corn and soy-based highly processed foods that are loaded with salt, fat, and sugar, and low in any whole nutrition. These highly concentrated sources of nutrients are highly addictive, and have crowded out the inclusion of healthier fare, including fresh fruits, vegetables and whole grains. It certainly is a huge change from what nature intended.

Nutrition experts used to say that Americans had the "best diet in the world"—but what we really have is biggest caloric intake in the world, and those calories are often devoid of nutrients. Thus, in our wealthy western society, nutrient deficiencies are widespread, including iron, calcium, and B vitamins. In addition, vitamin D deficiency is now widespread because our main source of vitamin D is sunlight, and many of us either don't go outside anymore, or we slather on the sunscreen before venturing out, which inhibits our skin's ability to manufacture vitamin D. These nutrient deficiencies, along with excesses of fat, salt, and sugar, have resulted in a massive increase in chronic diseases, including obesity, diabetes, high blood pressure, heart disease, cancer, arthritis–and depression. Many studies have shown the benefit of great nutrition on mood, including the moods of depressed children, as well as men in prison. We need healthy whole food if we expect to have healthy bodies and minds.

Let's look at some specific areas of focus:

Inflammation

A highly processed diet seems to contribute to what we call inflammation—the production of chemicals in the body that irritate the tissues and promote wear, tear, and aging. Some inflammation is good—it can help to mobilize your immune cells when needed, e.g. to fight infection. Too much inflammation however is like a forest-fire out of control—it burns up the healthy forest.

Some research has shown that the chemicals in the body associated with inflammation, including IL-6 and TNF-a, have a negative impact on the brain and can inhibit production of healthy new brain cells; they also stimulate the production of the stress hormone cortisol. These changes are felt to increase the risk for depression[71]. You can reduce any unnecessary inflammation by eating whole, unprocessed foods—fruits, veggies, whole unprocessed grains, legumes, and fish which are high in antioxidants—and by avoiding fried, greasy, and processed foods (regular exercise, maintaining a healthy weight, reducing your stress levels, and avoiding tobacco also reduce inflammation). Reducing your intake of animal food will also reduce inflammation, and some studies have suggested that the incidence of depression is lower in people who follow a vegetarian diet.

Carbohydrates and Protein

Carbohydrates (aka "carbs") are precursors to serotonin, one of multiple neurotransmitters (chemical messengers) in the brain; serotonin helps to calm our frazzled mind. In fact although not completely understood, it is felt that most of the commonly used prescription anti-depressants work by increasing serotonin in the brain. You can help to boost your body's own serotonin supply by including lots of healthy whole grain carbs in your diet, including quinoa, whole oats, barley, and millet. Avoid refined carbs like white flours and sugars, which are mostly devoid of micronutrients and also contribute to unnecessary inflammation in the body.

Healthy proteins are also part of a brain-smart diet. Protein foods like turkey, chicken, and tuna are rich in the amino acid tyrosine, and tyrosine helps to boost neurotransmitters in the brain such as dopamine and norepinephrine. Norepinephrine helps us to feel alert, and dopamine is sometimes called the neurotransmitter of happiness or positive emotions. Most Americans get more protein than they need, especially from animal sources, so you probably don't need to worry about any protein deficiency in your diet. However, some studies suggest a lower risk of depression in people who eat a vegetarian or plant-based diet, so shifting from animal to plant sources of protein may be beneficial for your mood. The average person needs about 0.4 grams of protein per pound of body weight.

Healthy Fats
The kind of fat that we eat also seems to play a major role in mood. Here's a little background: The essential fatty acids (EFAs) are polyunsaturated fats that

our bodies cannot make for themselves; we must obtain them from our diets. The two main classes of EFAs are the omega-6 and the omega-3 fatty acids. The omega-3 fats, EPA and DHA, are those famous fats everyone hears about these days that are found primarily in fish and fish oils; a precursor to this fat known as ALA, is found in certain plants including flaxseed, walnuts, and dark green leafy vegetables. Our body has to convert ALA to EPA/DHA, though some people are genetically not able to do this—they must rely instead on fish oil or algae-derived EPA/DHA for preformed EPA/DHA. Omega-3 fats are important for the healthy functioning of many of the cells in our body, especially our brain cells; they work in part by reducing the production of inflammatory chemicals.

What about those omega-6 fats? They include the common oils in our diet, like soybean and corn oil, and they are widespread in our food supply. In fact, look at the label of just about any baked or processed food you might find in the grocery story, and you're likely to see an omega-6 oil on the nutrition label. When consumed in reasonable amounts, omega-6 oils are an essential and healthy part of our diet. However, when they are processed (ie, turned into trans-fats) or when they are consumed in excess, they may contribute to the production of inflammatory chemicals in the body.

Why is all of this important to your mood? It's because the omega-6 and the omega-3 oils "duke it out" in our cells to get center stage; the more omega-6 fats you eat, or the less omega-3 you eat, the more the omega-3s are crowded out. In fact, our consumption of omega-6 oils has soared over the past century (think "french fries)–100 years ago, omega-6 oils accounted for about one-half percent of the total calories in our diet; these days, about ten percent of our calories come from omega-6 fats. Add that to a lack of omega-3 foods in your fridge, and you may be setting yourself up for an omega-6:omega-3 imbalance or an omega-3 deficiency state. And, those omega-3s are needed for the healthy functioning of cell membranes, especially those in your brain. They may also improve the production and func-tioning of neurotransmitters like dopamine, which have a strong impact on mood. Some studies suggest that they reduce anxiety, depression, and violent behav-ior; they also reduce the risk of suicide[72]. Fish oils may also improve literacy, attention, and standardized test scores. And, they seem to reduce inflammation and the stress response in the body to boot. Mess with those omega-3s in your diet, and you may notice that your mood tanks a bit too[73]. In fact, researchers have noticed that the incidence of depression is higher in countries with low intakes of fish[74].

So what's the bottom line here? Although the data is still early, we strongly encourage anyone with depres-sion or a tendency towards depression to eat fish on a regular basis (translation: at least 3 servings per week), or take fish oil supplements–roughly 1,000 mg of EPA/ DHA per day as a baseline (don't forget to look at the label of your supplement to see exactly how much DHA and EPA is in each capsule); some people may need more than this to have an impact on mood, but we recommend that you speak with your personal physician first. If you're one who tends toward fish-breath with these supplements, try storing them in the freezer—this can reduce side effects for some people.

Vitamins, Herbs and Other Supplements That Can Support Your Mood

• B vitamins

The B vitamins seem to play an important role in mood, especially vitamins B6, B12, and folic acid. These vitamins are needed for the production of several important neurotransmitters, including serotonin, dopamine, and norepinephrine, and low blood levels are associated with depression[75]. In addition, those people with low blood levels may not respond fully to anti-depressant medication, or may be at higher risk for relapse of depression. It is not clear whether B vitamin deficiency actually leads to depression, or whether it is a marker for something else that affects mood; there is no definitive data yet showing that treatment with B vitamins reduces depression, though some early data suggests that folate may improve the response to antidepressant meds[76]. And, B vitamin deficiency is often widespread, especially in those who eat a poor diet and do not take any vitamin supplements. B12 deficiency is also widespread amongst the elderly. So although our understanding of B vitamins and mood is still incomplete, we recommend that you take a daily multivitamin or B-complex supplement; since adults over the age of 50 need more B12, if you are over 50, you should take a supplement designed for older adults. And, the B vitamins work in concert together, so it's best to take them as a complex, and not as individual supplements.

- **Vitamin D**

Vitamin D seems to play an important role in mood; it is needed for the synthesis of multiple neurotransmitters in the brain[77]. In the recent past, vitamin D deficiency has become a widespread problem for several reasons. Throughout history, humans have relied on sun exposure for their vitamin D. When the sun hits our skin, a vitamin D precursor is activated and sent to the liver where the conversion into active vitamin D begins. In the winter months, when the sun is less strong in the sky and we stay indoors more, blood levels of vitamin D tend to drop, sometimes to very low levels. In addition, many of us spend little time out of doors now (think: video games), or if we do, we slather on the sunscreen, which prevents our skin from making much vitamin D. And finally, as we age, our skin becomes much less efficient at manufacturing the vitamin D that we need to be healthy. The result? Vitamin D deficiency is now felt to be an epidemic problem. And, while we used to think of vitamin D as primarily a bone health nutrient, researchers have found that vitamin D is important for every tissue in the body, including your brain[78]—hence the probable connection with mood. In fact, if you're one of those people who experience depression during the winter months, also known as Seasonal Affective

Disorder or "SAD," you may be experiencing a vitamin D deficiency (many people become vitamin D deficient in the winter months when the suns rays are less strong and we spend less time out of doors). Some people with SAD improve with light therapy, which may also work by raising your vitamin D blood level. Most Americans should be taking a daily vitamin D supplement; aim for 1,000 to 2,000 units of vitamin D3 every day (foods like dairy products are *not* felt to be reliable sources of vitamin D). Talk with your doctor first before taking a vitamin D supplement if you have kidney disease or other chronic illness. You might also want to consider getting your vitamin D blood level checked; an *optimal* level is probably above 50 ng/ml.

- **St. John's Wort**

St .John's Wort is an herb that has been used medicinally for over 2,000 years to treat emotional disorders. Of all the alternative therapies that have been tested for depression and anxiety, St. John's Wort seems to be the most effective. It works much like prescription anti-depressants by raising levels of serotonin, dopamine, and norepinephrine in the brain; it may impact other neurotransmitters as well. Studies suggest that St. John's Wort probably works as well as prescription antidepressants for people with mild to moderate depression, though it often has fewer side effects than prescription meds[79]. The main concern with St. John's Wort is that it can cause potentially dangerous interactions with numerous medications, including Plavix, oral contraceptives, and drugs used for organ-transplant patients. It is *very* important that you speak with your doctor before starting St. John's Wort, especially if you take any prescription meds. The active ingredients in St. John's Wort are hypericin and hyperforin; most products are standardized to 0.3% hypericin and are taken as 300 mg three times daily. You should not take any prescription antidepressants while taking St. John's Wort, as this can lead to dangerously elevated levels of serotonin in the blood and brain.

- **SAMe**

SAMe is an amino acid-like chemical that has been found to reduce pain and improve mood. It is made in our tissues, and also obtained from protein foods. It seems to have an influence on cell communication in the brain and also increases norepinephrine and dopamine levels; it has an impact on our serotonin levels as well. Several studies have shown that SAMe can be as effective at improving mood as some of the prescription antidepressant medications[80]. The main problem with SAMe is that it is very expensive, and the quality of products available over the counter may be poor. SAMe can also raise blood serotonin levels just like St. John's Wort, so it should not be taken with any prescription antidepressants.

If you wish to try SAMe to help your mood, talk with your doctor. Typical doses used for depression are 400-600 mg twice daily. There are several forms of SAMe that are on the market; if you decide to try it, look for the butane-disulfonate salt form of SAMe, which is the most bioavailable and also the most stable.

- **5-HTP and L-tryptophan**

As mentioned above, serotonin is a key neurotransmitter in the regulation of mood, and many prescription anti-depressant medications work by increasing serotonin levels in the brain. Serotonin is manufactured in the body from the amino acids tryptophan and 5-hydroxytryptophan (5-HTP): tryptophan is converted to 5-HTP, and 5-HTP is then converted into serotonin. There is some data to suggest that both of these supplements may improve mood[81]. The main concern with them, however, is safety; in 1989 a syndrome known as Eosinophilia-Myalgia Syndrome (EMS) was identified in more than 1500 people who used L-tryptophan, and 37 deaths were reported. Most of the people with EMS had taken an L-tryptophan supplement from a specific manufacturer in Japan, so the syndrome may have been caused by a contaminant in this specific product. However, the definitive cause of EMS was not identified, so the FDA removed all L-tryptophan supplements from the market in the US. L-tryptophan became available again several years later, but some experts still caution against using it. 5-HTP has not been linked to EMS, but some experts are still concerned about its safety. We do not recommend using either of these products first line for depression, but should you decide to try them, please speak with your doctor first. We also recommend that you subscribe to the testing lab ConsumerLab to choose a top-notch product (see below for more information). And finally, 5-HTP and tryptophan can raise blood serotonin levels just like St. John's Wort or SAMe, so they should not be taken with any prescription antidepressants.

- **Inositol**

Inositol is an essential component of cell membranes in the brain; it seems to have an impact on mood by improving cell communication. Some evidence from short-term studies suggests that inositol does help to relieve depression, panic disorder, anxiety, and obsessive-compulsive disorder much like prescription antidepressant or anti-anxiety medications[82]; longer studies are needed to assess the long-term efficacy and safety of this supplement. Inositol may interact with prescription medications, especially mood stabilizers, and there is also some concern that it may induce mania in people with bipolar depression, so talk with your doctor before considering inositol. The doses used in studies for depression and other mood disorders range from 12-18 grams per day; its effects seem to wear off as soon as it is discontinued. Inositol can cause some side effects like headaches, fatigue, and nausea, but overall it does appear to be a safe supplement and is usually pretty-well tolerated; long-term safety data are unavailable, however.

- **Probiotics**

Probiotics such as lactobacilli are "friendly" bacteria that line the intestinal tract; they live in balance with other bacteria like E. coli which can cause harm, and they help to keep these "unfriendly" bacteria in check. There is intriguing evidence that a reduction in healthy bacteria in the gut, coupled with a rise in harmful bacteria, can increase the risk of depression[83]. There seem to be several pathways by which this occurs: harmful bacteria may communicate with the central nervous system and negatively impact mood; harmful bacteria may also consume nutrients in the gut that are needed for healthy mood, including B vitamins; and harmful bacteria may increase inflammation in the gut, which can then increase the risk for mood disorders. What leads to a deficiency of healthy bacteria in the first place? Antibiotic usage kills off healthy bacteria; poor diet and chronic stress also seem to have a negative impact. If you want to try probiotics to improve your mood, be sure to get a product that has been tested for purity; probiotics (as well as all other herbs and supplements) are not regulated by the FDA. See below for more information on supplement purity and safety.

• **Other supplements**

Multiple other herbs and supplements have been used to reduce anxiety and improve mood, though definitive data is still preliminary. These include ginkgo, glutamine, lavender, lemon balm, passionflower, skullcap, saffron, theanine, and turmeric. Kava is also widely used for anxiety, but there are numerous reports of liver damage, at times severe, in people taking kava. We encourage you to do your research and talk with your doctor before taking any herb or supplement.

Choosing High Quality Supplements

While the FDA strictly regulates prescription medications, it does not regulate any of the over-the-counter supplements found in pharmacies and health food stores, including vitamins and herbs; when you purchase a supplement, you are not guaranteed that the bottle contains a product that is pure, effective, or safe. The supplement you purchase may also not contain 100% of the claimed amount of vitamins, herbal constituents, etc. In addition, products that are imported from other areas of the world such as Asia and India may be contaminated with heavy metals and/or prescription drugs. Therefore the onus of finding a good product falls on you, the consumer. This can be a critical issue, especially if you are taking something that is potentially toxic, or that may interfere with other medications or supplements you are taking. So, what can you do to educate yourself about this?

- If you use any over-the-counter supplements on a regular basis, we strongly encourage you to subscribe to www.consumerlab.com ($29.95/yr); this is an independent testing lab that provides information about the purity and quality of many brand name products on the market.
- Look for products that have the designation "USP" or "NF/GMP"; this suggests that they have undergone some evaluation of their purity and have passed muster (manufacturers submit to this on a voluntary basis).

- Look for reliable information on medical websites; WebMD is a good one, as are most of the websites at academic universities. Also, the Office of Dietary Supplements at the NIH is excellent; their website is http:// dietary-supplements.info.nih.gov.

-

Key points of this chapter:
- **Your food, your mood—a healthy diet plays a big role in your brain health, including your mood. Dump the junk and embrace a whole foods lifestyle.**
- **Eat fish at least several times a week, or take fish oil capsules every day.**
- **Take a vitamin D supplement; get your blood level checked and adjust your dose according to your blood level.**
- **Take a B-complex or multivitamin tablet every day (most multivitamins contain a full B-complex).**
- **Consider St. John's Wort, SAMe, 5-HTP, or probiotics—but talk with your doctor first.**
- **If you choose to take herbs or other supplements, subscribe to www.con-sumerlab.com to help you identify quality products.**

Chapter 10.

Challenging the Paradigm

We've spent a lot of this book talking about things that you can do to help yourself or the person you know who's suffering from depression. At a certain point, though, it's fair to ask—it may be that depression is everyone's problem, and that individuals and their support networks can accomplish a lot proactively, but isn't treating the people who have it ultimately a job for professionals?

In many cases, yes—but it's also important to understand that mental health professionals face their own set of obstacles when it comes to adapting their practices to the new science of exercise and depression.

For those professionals—psychiatrists and psychologists, individual, marriage and family counselors and others—the major hurdle to introducing exercise into the standard treatment regime for depression has always been acceptance.

A 1996 study found that, "even though many psychotherapists believe in the therapeutic value of exercise, only approximately 10 percent recommended exercise for their clients."[84] With the additional research published since then, and the arrival of what ought to be the conclusion of the scientific debate about the mood-elevating effects of exercise, we hope and believe that acceptance among mental health professionals of exercise as an adjunctive treatment for depression will increase. There is no longer any logical reason it shouldn't.

Of course, there's no logical reason why Wile E. Coyote keeps returning unscathed after falling off cliff after cliff while hunting the Roadrunner in all those Warner Brothers cartoons. Like the famous Mr. Coyote, the medical establishment at times appears impervious to all outside forces.

అశ

Setting aside questions of logic for the moment, a second major hurdle remains for mental health professionals who might be inclined to adopt exercise (or for that matter, other mind-body approaches) as part of their standard treatment plan for depression—a deficit of expertise.

Many mental health professionals exercise, but few have ever developed a program of exercise for someone else, and fewer still are certified professional trainers. By the same token, many professional trainers and physical education specialists are knowledgeable in the area of sports psychology, but few are licensed mental health professionals.

There are a couple of basic options for mental health professionals who are ready to begin using exercise as part of their treatment program for depressed patients. One is to educate themselves about how to create and monitor the progress of an exercise program for their patients. Another is to seek out an exercise professional who is willing and able to act as the therapist's partner in coaching patients through the development of an individualized exercise program.

For counselors who are interested in incorporating exercise into their own program of treatment for depression, some excellent resources are available. In particular, *Working It Out: Using Exercise in Psychotherapy* by Kate F. Hays (American Psychological Association, 1999) is the authoritative manual for mental health professionals who decide to make exercise an integral part of their practice. Clinical psychologist Hays employed sports psychology in her practice for 25 years and *Working It Out* is a veritable instruction manual for a psychology practice incorporating exercise as treatment. Chapter titles include "The Body-Mind Connection," "Choosing Exercise As A Therapeutic Tool" and "The Psychological Benefits of Exercise With Specific Populations," and the appendices include a development plan for practitioners and a set of suggested questions for interviewing patients about their exercise experiences, attitudes, abilities and preferences.

Another helpful resource is a 1996 article in which W.E. Sime offered this concise "starting point" set of guidelines for practitioners:[85]

1. Explore the client's exercise history to determine current exercise habits and past experiences in order to identify enjoyable activities critical to program adherence.

2. Participate in initial exercise sessions to serve as a model for appropriate client behavior.

3. Educate the client about the potential physical and mental health benefits of exercise as a commitment enhancement procedure.

4. Consider options to make exercise functional, such as commuting to work by walking, jogging, or biking or including home chores in the prescription.

5. Take advantage of the client's environment (e.g., parks, lakes, fitness trails, home equipment) in facilitating exercise activity.

6. Help the client choose enjoyable activities from a broad spectrum of choices.

7. Prescribe the type, duration, frequency, and intensity of the exercise program in terms of the client's current level of conditioning. Clinicians who are not trained or experienced in exercise physiology are advised to seek the assistance of a local specialist who can supervise the ongoing prescription process.

8. Attempt to facilitate exercise within a positive social milieu.

9. Assist the client to develop behavioral self-control strategies (e.g., behavioral contracting, stimulus

control, positive reinforcement) to improve program adherence.

10. Prepare the client for recidivism and reinitiation using relapse prevention strategies.

The second bullet above may be a new point of resistance for some practitioners. *You want me to what? Exercise with my patient?* For some this will undoubtedly feel like a very foreign and/or impractical idea, but it's more than just a cutting-edge concept—it's an approach to treatment that a number of professionals have already begun proving out in their own practices.

For example, Washington, D.C. counselor Jane Cibel has her patients walk on a treadmill during therapy sessions.[86] The licensed clinical social worker is also a certified personal trainer who conducts her practice out of her basement, which contains both a standard therapist's office set-up with a desk and couches on one side of the room, and a full home gym complete with treadmill, workout bench and free weights on the other. Cibel is a true believer in the therapeutic value of her approach, declaring that "You can restructure your brain with exercise."

Of course, not every mental health professional will feel comfortable or qualified to take such a holistic approach. Those who prefer to stay on what is for them more familiar territory will want to follow Sime's recommendation number seven and seek out collaborators—exercise professionals who are interested in partnering with them to treat and coach patients. Between the proliferation of personal trainers and physical therapists, and the steady growth of the field of sports psychology, we're confident that most motivated mental health professionals could find suitable collaborators to help them incorporate exercise into their practices.

The biggest hurdle for practitioners, then, remains the simplest: acceptance. Ultimately, we can only rely on the desire of counseling professionals to help their patients, and on their willingness to challenge the existing paradigm of depression treatment with new and therefore still unconventional wisdom. The evolution in thinking about treatment modes is profound, but the logic behind it couldn't be simpler. If you sprain your ankle, the doctor's first recommendation is usually physical therapy. With what we know today, it should be no different for depression.

అ‑ఌ

We've been fairly tough here on the medical establishment—so now, let's also make sure to be fair as well.

In that category of "wouldn't it be nice if…" we offer the following: wouldn't it be nice if health care professionals were free to simply provide the care they know will serve their patients best, regardless of insurance policy or government program rules?

But that is not the reality we live in. The American insurance-based health care system is full of limitations not just for patients but for doctors. Treatments are authorized by insurance companies and state health plans based not just on their effectiveness, but on their familiarity and their efficiency. The core purpose of the insurance industry is, after all, risk management. If there is one question none of these folks wants to hear on their voice mail, it's "You're paying for *what*?!"

There is in fact a substantial bias in our health care system (and the policy-makers who stand behind it) in favor of man-made, hi-tech solutions and against natural remedies. Much as we have come to view humans as master of the earth we inhabit, we are often tempted to view ourselves as masters of our own bodies. We invest such unwavering confidence in the science underlying our medical system that if something is wrong with us, we look immediately to "advanced" (i.e. manufactured) tools—typically prescription drugs and medical technology—to solve the problem. In our hubris, we have adopted our own cleverest inventions as our first and often only resort, and viewed approaches that diverge from the slow-to-evolve conventional wisdom of the Western medical establishment with immediate suspicion.

That same conventional wisdom dominates the thinking of policy-makers, health systems and insurers even today—witness the recent study that showed psychiatrists today receive higher reimbursement from insurers for medication-only appointments than for psy-chotherapy appointments.[87] Most insurers and health plan administrators are reflexively skeptical of forms of treatment that don't involve deploying man-made chemicals or technology. And because they rely on the medical professionals working within the system to sup-ply the technical expertise they generally lack, it will fall primarily on those same practitioners to bring about an evolution of the system's perspective on the value of exercise as a treatment for depression.

What these practitioners and the system within which they operate all need to appreciate is that the mental health care establishment is failing patients to-day, by failing to adopt exercise as a standard mode of treatment for depression. The science is already there. What we're waiting for now is the system—counselors, doctors, insurers, employers and policy-makers—to catch up.

In the meantime, the ones who are suffering be-cause of our health care system's failure to adapt are the people whom it was created to help and support—the patients. This is more than unfortunate, and more than a shame. It's a tragedy.

෨᳇෨

Key points in this chapter:

- **Mental health professionals face their own set of obstacles when it comes to** incorporating exercise (as well as other alternative modes of treatment) to their practices.

- Acceptance of these alternative methods as valid modes of treatment is increasing but not yet widespread.

- Expertise is another barrier—although more and more mental health practitioners are learning from or partnering with exercise professionals to incorporate exercise into their practices.

- *Working It Out: Using Exercise in Psychotherapy* by Kate F. Hays is the authoritative manual for mental health professionals who decide to make exercise part of their practice.

- The risk management orientation of the insurance industry is another obstacle, creating financial barriers and encouraging a quick-fix approach that relies more on chemical remedies than potential alternatives.

- The tragedy of the situation is that the ones who are suffering because of our health care system's failure to adapt are the people whom it was created to help and support—the patients.

Chapter 11.

The Revolution Starts Now

We've talked about the specific ways that you can help yourself or the person you know and care about who is depressed. And we've talked about the evolution in thinking that our medical establishment needs to undergo for that help to become more available. Before we close, though, we want to draw your attention back to the bigger picture again for a moment.

Let's start by going back to the numbers. One in 10 adults suffers from depression. Four in five people with it or related illnesses don't seek treatment. More than $13 billion is spent annually on antidepressant medications taken by, in some states, up to 16 percent of the population. A hundred billion dollars—that's $100,000,000,000—is spent every year on psychological care. And depression costs American businesses $44 billion a year in lost productivity.

Can there be any question that depression is one of the major public health issues of the 21st century? We don't think so.

Depression affects millions of lives, costs the government and private insurers billions in health care expenses, and burdens private employers everywhere with lost productivity due to a common and often highly curable condition. The fact that we're still squeamish about talking about mental illness and react skeptically to new treatment methods that diverge from the old conventional wisdom only ensures that unnecessary suffering continues.

Our health care system's response to the problem to date has been to continue giving in to our society's preference for quick fixes and rely more and more on man-made chemical solutions rather than looking deeper into ourselves. That position is no longer viable. We have known for years that exercise elevates mood. Now we understand much more about how and why. The science is there, but the system hasn't caught up yet.

Or at least, the system as a whole hasn't caught up yet. Some within it, however, are starting to. A quiet revolution is beginning to take hold, and it's coming from where all revolutions start—the street. Individuals taking new ideas driven by new science and—quite literally—running with them.

ॐ⋅ॐ

Dr. Michael Conner is a clinical psychologist whose practice in Bend, Oregon is on leading edge of a wave of change in the field of mental health.

"I'm so convinced of the benefits of exercise that I'm actually putting a gym in a separate room in my office," says Conner. "I'm going to introduce people to some very simple exercises, particularly for patients who are afraid to get a gym membership or are intimidated by the equipment or think it's going to be too difficult."[88]

By introducing his patients to the benefits of exercise in the safe, controlled environment of his psychology practice, Dr. Conner significantly increases his patients' odds of overcoming obstacles such as lack of motivation or experience with exercise. Still, he recognizes the hurdles clearly: "It's not a promise for everybody," he says. "And that's what I tell my patients." But he goes on to tell them "If you don't want to be on drugs your whole life, exercise may be the key."

Conner came to the conclusion that he should integrate exercise into his psychology in part because of his familiarity with Babyak and Blumenthal's Duke University study. He took special note of the six-month outcomes, which saw the positive effects of exercise treatment alone endure longer and better than those of medication or medication plus exercise. "People who continue to exercise have lower relapse rates."[89]

❧❧

One gets the sense that Dr. Conner doesn't necessarily consider himself a revolutionary. But the truth is that he and those of his peers who are not just recognizing the truth that years of scientific study has brought us around to, but acting on it and evolving their approach to patient care, are the agents of change who will drive the transformation our health care system needs to undergo.

The question is, who will join them?

Revolutions may start in the streets, but they are ultimately won in boardrooms and seats of government. They are won when eyes that have been shut fall open to the new reality before them—eyes belonging to those with their hands on the levers of power. In this case, the eyes and hands in question belong to employers and insurers and state and federal health policy-makers.

We don't discount the possibility that individuals moving at the highest circles of power in and around America's health care system might behave in an altruistic way. Many are strongly supportive of their employees, customers and constituents, and genuinely concerned about patient outcomes. But we're also realistic. Whether an employer's business is large or small, their success depends on the productivity of their employees. Whether a health care institution or program or insurer is for-profit or non-profit or government-run, they want to fund treatments that work, and all else being equal, they want to fund treatments that have a rational cost-benefit ratio.

They want maximum bang for the buck. Who wouldn't?

So let's quit the emotional appeals for a minute and talk in terms the bottom-line folks understand: money. Think back to the data we cited in the introduction about the $44 billion in lost productivity attributable to depression. Think back to the $13.5 billion spent every year for antidepressants. Think back to the study we talked about in which patients who had been on prescription antidepressants for an average of four years with nominal effect showed marked improvement after just three weeks of regular exercise. Now imagine that the results of this study held for every person in America dealing with depression.

And then, do the math. Add $44 billion in lost productivity plus $13.5 billion in antidepressant costs to get $57.5 billion, and then multiply by the four years the people in Craft's study spent barely getting by with prescription medications. That's $230 billion—the bulk of it paid by insurers and employers, and then passed on to consumers—in lost productivity and spending on prescription medications that have been scientifically proven to be not as effective a treatment for depression as three weeks of regular exercise.

The conclusion is clear: paying for a depressed patient/employee to go to a personal trainer for a month before resorting to antidepressants isn't just a good medical decision—it's a good business decision.

∂∾∾

Meanwhile, signs are increasing that the revolution may be ready to spread beyond the offices of a few innovative practitioners.

In 1996, the Surgeon General's Report on Physical Activity and Health declared that "physical activity appears to relieve symptoms of depression" and that "regular physical activity may reduce the risk of developing depression, although further research is needed on this topic."[90] (It will be interesting to see what the next Surgeon General's report on this topic says, considering the research that's been done since 1996.) In 1999, the American Psychological Association issued a report describing exercise as "an effective but underused treatment" for depression.[91] Today its Web site includes an entire page trumpeting exercise as "an effective, cost-effective treatment for depression" and "a third successful alternative" to psychotherapy and prescription medication.[92] Several years ago, the handful of therapists like Keith Johnsgard who incorporated exercise into their practices were viewed as oddballs, but today the famously conservative *Wall Street Journal* turns out a fresh article exploring their growing numbers every year or so.[93]

Meanwhile, psychiatrists—who go through the additional years of medical training necessary to become a psychiatrist precisely so that they can write prescriptions for their patients—have perhaps understandably been slower to warm up to the idea of exercise as a viable alternative. The American Psychiatric Association has made no official comment about the medicinal value of exercise, and its guidelines for treating depression still mention only medication and psychotherapy.[94] As *Spark*'s Dr. Ratey explains,

"...the allure of the magic pill is powerful, and it takes a long time to overturn attitudes. Just ask T. Byram Karasu, who was in charge of the American Psychiatric Association's work group on major depressive disorders. He pushed to get the APA to formally adopt exercise in its treatment guidelines for depression and suggested that psychiatrists tell every patient to walk three to five miles a day or do some other type of vigorous exercise. The APA balked, presumably because, while most doctors acknowledge the anecdotal evidence that exercise improves mood, they say there isn't enough scientific evidence."[95]

Along the same lines, an e-mailed "Depression & Anxiety Health Alert" from the Johns Hopkins School of Medicine suggests "What To Do When Your Antidepressant Doesn't Work"—the options offered being switching medications or increasing doses, without a single mention of any treatment strategy for depression other than more and/or different prescription drugs.[96] In fact, the doctor the APA commonly refers inquiries about exercise to—California psychiatrist Dr. James Lake—is very direct about the inherent bias of his peers. "Because of collective professional values and financial interests of academic psychiatry," he says, "research priorities have almost exclusively targeted psychopharmacology."[97]

What's true in America is not necessarily the case elsewhere, though. The United Kingdom in particular appears to be ahead of the U.S. on this count. In 2005, the British Mental Health Foundation reported the "mounting evidence that a supervised exercise programme could treat mild to moderate depression as well as drugs," and provided clinical guidelines for the use of exercise as a treatment for depression.[98] And while the same report found that only 5 percent of UK doctors recommended exercise as a treatment option, and that 78 percent had prescribed an anti-depressant in the past three years despite believing that an alternative treatment might have been more appropriate, it also found that younger doctors were more likely to recommend exercise, and called for the British government to invest 20 million pounds in "developing and promoting" exercise as treatment for mild to moderate depression.

It's vital that mental health professionals take the lead in the movement to change how we approach treating depression, and it's heartening to see signs that their efforts are beginning to gain traction both in the U.S. and in the U.K. Their task is a huge one, though, because they are working to overcome not just decades of conventional wisdom about treating depression, but very well-organized and funded promotional campaigns aimed at keeping patients and doctors focused on anti-depressants as the first and best remedy for depression. Prescription medications have hundreds of millions of dollars in research and advertising money behind them, and all exercise has is a small cadre of mental health professionals trying to talk their patients into getting up off the couch.

ॐॐ

Education of mental health professionals about the benefits of exercise for treating depression is vital. A transformation in the thinking of corporate leaders about how they want their employees treated for depression is essential. But even that combination of forces is unlikely to be enough without a nudge from the political system. Policy-makers must also take up the cause.

Why should they care? Well, if ten percent of their constituents being affected by the same health problem isn't enough, how about this: a study published by the World Health Organization last year declared depression to be "a more disabling condition than angina, arthritis, asthma and diabetes" and found that depression substantially worsened patient outcomes for people who also had other health problems. In the words of study leader Dr. Somnath Chatterji: "These results indicate the urgency of addressing depression as a public health priority to reduce disease burden and disability, and improve the overall health of populations."[99]

The pitfalls of legislating this sort of change are evident, though. In California, for example, Assemblyman Lloyd Levine introduced a bill in 2008 to require companies that bid on large state contracts and have more than 10 employees to promote healthy lifestyles. Companies could do so through a variety of methods, including subsidizing health club memberships.

The response from industry was indignant: "Why are we putting the responsibility on businesses?" groused a spokesperson for the National Federation of Independent Businesses. "It's individuals who make decisions about their lifestyles." You know the answer to that question, and Levine does too, citing "numerous studies that document loss of productivity resulting from conditions such as asthma and diabetes [and depression] that could be prevented or mitigated with exercise." Employees who exercise are both healthier and more productive employees.

Levine is realistic about the chances of his bill making it beyond the conceptual stage, acknowledging that it's unlikely to become law. "But my hope," he concludes, "is that it will start a discussion."[100] It's a discussion we need to have if the quiet revolution surrounding how we treat depression is to continue gaining momentum, and we need to have it everywhere from therapists' offices to board rooms to the halls of government. This cause has everything it ought to need to catch fire—a massive public health problem, and an inexpensive solution with good science behind it. All that's required for this revolution to succeed is for a group of committed advocates to stand up and demand to be heard.

☙❧

Key points in this chapter:

- **Measured in terms of costs to society, depression is one of the major public health issues of the 21st century.**
- **Our health care system's response has been to perpetuate the quick fix mentality and rely on man-made chemical solutions rather than looking deeper into ourselves.**
- **At the same time, though, a quiet revolution is underway, led by mental health practitioners who are willing to break from the pack and embrace exercise and other alternative modes of treatment for depression.**
- **This movement needs, and should receive, support from industry leaders and policy-makers, not just because the science is there (although it is), but because exercise and related modes of treatment are also more cost-effective. That is, paying for a depressed patient/employee to go to a personal trainer for a month before resorting to antidepressants isn't just a good medical decision—it's a good business decision.**
- **Mainstream voices are catching on as well, as the Surgeon General, the American Psychological Association,**

and even the **Wall Street Journal** have begun writing more and more favorably about the proven mental health benefits of exercise.

- **Resistance remains among some mental health professionals, but the tide may be turning, especially if business leaders and policy-makers can be motivated to take up the cause.**

Chapter 12.
The Ultimate Prescription

If you've read this far, it's at least in part because you understand what's at stake.

You understand that depression is one of the major health issues of our time, that it is literally everyone's problem. And hopefully you understand a little more than you did when you started this book about the history and science of exercise as a remedy for depression.

But you've probably read this far mostly because, like us, your life or the life of someone you care about has been touched by depression—and you want to help.

As we said in the introduction, we wrote *The Ultimate Prescription* for two reasons. First, we wanted to offer hope and motivation to people suffering from depression and their loved ones. And second, we wanted to educate everyone involved with our mental health care system—patients and therapists, doctors and hospitals, insurers and employers, opinion leaders and policy-makers—about the new science that can and should revolutionize the way we treat depression in America and around the world.

The stakes could not be higher. Millions of people are affected either directly or indirectly by depression. As a society, we spend billions of dollars a year for treatments that both expensive and too often ineffective. And those costs are inevitable passed back to employers (and consumers) and government health programs (and taxpayers).

We simply cannot afford to cling to the conventional wisdom of the past when confronted by scientific realities that demand a change in our thinking. Exercise is an effective treatment for depression. We know this. Endorphins are most likely the mechanism for the beneficial effects of exercise on depression. We know this, too. We also know that nutrition, supplements, and mind-body strategies can have a major impact on mental well-being and happiness.

At this point, what we don't know yet is how long it will take our health care system to catch up to this new reality, and how many lives will be damaged or how much productivity lost as a result of a reluctance to adapt to new information. Yes, there are hurdles, but none that people of good will and imagination and commitment can't overcome.

Not just that person you know, but millions of people out there need your help. To paraphrase an old saying, all that's necessary for a bad outcome is for peo-ple of good will to do nothing. The outcome for millions suffering from depression—family, friends, patients, col-leagues, employees, clients and constituents—is now in your hands.

Afterword

by John D. Winters

This book is ultimately about a journey that each of us must, in the end, take alone.

All of us face doubts and fears related to our abilities and what we are capable of. One of the most essential elements of this book is the need for action on the part of the individual. Not all of the ideas presented here will help to motivate a person dealing with depression to be proactive. But what I have hoped from the outset is that increasing awareness of a variety of different ways—including exercise—to affect change in your own or someone else's life can make a real difference in peoples' lives.

The very idea of change is so challenging that many choose not to try. Part of what led me to want to write this book is two personal experiences that allowed me to change my direction, attitude and life forever.

In November 1976, I was at the edge of death from cerebral edema, lying in a hypothermic coma in the Himalayas. When the doctor arrived, I had no pulse. It was obvious that I was going to need to make a choice.

Fighting for my life turned out to be the hardest thing I have ever done. I remember hearing the doctor asking me to give the injection a chance to work, to try and wake again. A moment of consciousness to make the decision of your life. Observing this scene from afar in the desolate mountainous valley, I vividly remember making the choice to fight, and the days that followed were driven by my overwhelming desire to live. All of the efforts of the doctor and my companions on the trek, all of their caring encouragement to keep going would not have been enough to make it through the three days it took to reach the hospital without the desire I had within me, the choice I made to embrace the blessing that life is. I learned that day to cherish the opportunity our lives provide us; to give, to love, to enjoy and to appreciate each breath, and to remember that tomorrow might not come.

Making choices is never an easy process. Not all the avenues we choose during this journey result in the achievement of the goals we saw so clearly at the outset. It's like Reverend Mother said to Maria in *The Sound of Music*: "When God closes a door, he opens a window." Others have asked "how do you hold a moonbeam in your hand?" or "how do you keep a wave upon the sand?" The concepts might seem elusive, but the words ultimately illustrate the power of our mind to construct positive thoughts, and persist.

The other story that reflects a significant change in my life has to do with the experience I had as a young boy of being told by a fellow student that I had been adopted. After learning this at eight years old from someone other than my parents, I was confused and very angry. Lying in bed at night, crying into my pillow, that anger was directed at everyone, including my adoptive parents as well as the birth parents I never knew. You might be surprised how many years you can spend being angry and imagining every potential scenario about who your birth parents are, how and where they live, or if they are even alive. Eventually I came to understand that my adoptive parents had given me a great opportunity and began to truly hear them when they told me, repeatedly, "We choose you to be our son."

Some years later in middle school I remember reading in science class something about how little we humans use of our brain. I thought that if I could only use a little bit more than others, I could be smarter and successful. I'm sure that all of my fantasies and efforts in this pursuit were statistically fruitless. What I learned instead, over time, is that I must live in the moment, be positive, behave positively, and live by the values I believe in.

That's what this book is about, at its core—living fully, respecting the connection between mind and body, and considering what you can do to change your perspective about your ability to move to a happier state of being.

Tens of millions of people have a hard time getting up and becoming active, whether because of depression or some other issue. My greatest concern after watching people I care about struggle with depression is that this problem is so real and prevalent in our society. It's so important to equip ourselves with an understanding of the tools we can use to help ourselves and our loved ones to emerge from this awful darkness. I believe that if we don't take action, in the next 15 years depression will become "the silent pandemic."

For reasons we have discussed, the sociological environment will continue to make depression the disease that we fear most, even as science grants us new tools to combat it. The decoding of the human genome in 1992 was a major step forward toward curing many of the major health concerns of our time. The shock of 2025 may be the recognition that hundreds of millions of people in developed countries around the world are suffering from the same common, treatable condition: depression.

What each of us needs in the end is a torch to light the path before us. The light can come from a friend, a family member, or ourselves, but ultimately that light must be felt from within to be effective at altering your mood and motivating you to take the next step forward. In that endeavor, the most important things you can do are to help others, be compassionate, and give love to be loved.

"Namaste" is a Sanskrit greeting with many interpretations, but is commonly understood to mean something like "I honor the light within you." My greatest hope is that the ideas you take from our work may bring you happiness and joy on your journey. Namaste.

End Matter

Extensive research went into the creation of *The Ultimate Prescription*. There is a substantial amount of informative reading available on the subject of exercise and depression, much of which falls into one of three camps—highly detailed, academically-oriented papers, articles, and books; practical, patient/consumer-oriented guides to treating depression; and superficial (and not always 100% accurate) mass media coverage. *The Ultimate Prescription* purposely falls within none of these camps; our objective was to present the hard science in layman's terms and present it concisely and with a distinct argument behind it, i.e. this is important information for everyone from patients to doctors to health policy-makers to understand and act on.

In an effort to make this bibliography as useful as possible for those inclined to dig further into the topic, we have divided it into subject areas as follows: Clinical Studies, Meta-Analyses, Media Coverage and General Reference. Meta-Analyses are the several academic analyses that have been done in an attempt to aggregate the findings of multiple different studies examining the effectives of exercise (and sometimes other treatments) on depression (and sometimes other conditions). The other categories are hopefully self-explanatory.

Clinical Studies

Artal, Michael with Carl Sherman; "Exercise Against Depression"; *The Physician and Sportsmedicine* (1998), 26(10); retrieved online April 3, 2008 at http://www.physsportsmed.com/issues/1998/10Oct/artal.htm.

Babyak, Michael, James A. Blumenthal, Steve Herman, Parinda Khatri, Murali Doraiswamy, Kathleen Moore, Edward Craighead, Teri T. Baldewicz, K. Ranga Krishnan; "Exercise Treatment for Major Depression: Maintenance of Therapeutic Benefit at 10 Months"; *Psychosomatic Medicine* (2000) 62:633-638.

Blumenthal, J.A., M.A. Babyak, K.A. Moore, W.A. Craighead, S. Herman, P. Khatri, R. Waugh, M.A. Napolitano, P.M. Doraiswami, K.R. Krishnan; "Effects of exercise training on older adults with major depression"; *Archives of Internal Medicine* (1999), 159:2349-56.

Boecker, Henning, Till Sprenger, Mary E. Spilker, Gjermund Henriksen, Marcus Koeppenhoefer, Klaus J. Wagner, Michael Valet, Achim Berthele, Thomas R. Tolle; "The Runner's High: Opiodergic Mechanisms in the Human Brain"; *Cerebral Cortex*, February 21, 2008.

- Boecker study news release—"The myth of runner's high revisited with brain imaging"; University of Bonn news release; 3/3/08; retrieved online on 4/14/08 at http://www.

eurekalert.org/pub/releases/2008-03/uob-tmo030308.php.

Craft, Lynette L.; "Exercise and clinical depression: examining two psychological mechanisms"; *Psychology of Sport and Exercise* (2005) 6(2):151-171.

Dunn, Andrea L., Madhukar H. Trivedi, James B. Kampert, Camillia G. Clark, Heather O. Chambliss; "Exercise Treatment for Depression"; *American Journal of Preventative Medicine* (2005) 28:1.

Phillips, Wayne T., Michaela Kiernan, Abby C. King; "Physical Activity as a Nonpharmacological Treatment for Depression: A Review"; *Complementary Health Practice Review* (2003) 8:139-152

Meta-Analyses

Daley, Amanda J.; "Exercise therapy and mental health in clinical populations: is exercise therapy a worthwhile intervention?"; *Advances in Psychiatric Treatment* (2002) 8: 262-270.

Landers, Daniel M.; "The Influence of Exercise on Mental Health"; *President's Council on Physical Fitness and Sports Research Digest* Series 2, Number 12; December 1997; retrieved online on January 11, 2008 at http://www.fitness.gov/mentalhealth.htm.

Martinsen, E.W.; "Exercise and Depression"; International Journal of Sport and Exercise Psychology (2005) 3(4):469-483.

North, T. Christian, Penny McCullagh & Zung Vu Tran; "Effect of Exercise on Depression"; *Exercise and Sport Science Reviews* (1989), 18:379-415.

Penedo, Frank J. and Jason R. Dahn; "Exercise and Well-Being: A Review of Mental and Physical Health Benefits Associated With Physical Activity"; *Current Opinions in Psychiatry* (2005) 18(2): 189-193.

Steinberg, Hannah and Elizabeth A. Sykes; "Introduction to Symposium on Endorphins and Behavioural Processes; Review of Literature on Endorphins and Exercise"; *Pharmocology Biochemistry & Behaviour*, Vol. 23 (1985); pp. 857-862.

Tkachuk, Gregg A. and Garry L. Martin; "Exercise Therapy for Patients With Psychiatric Disorders: Research and Clinical Implications"; *Professional Psychology: Research and Practice* (1999), 30(3):275-282.

Media Coverage

"Acupuncture works on endorphins"; News In Science, ABC.net; retrieved online on April 22, 2008 at: http://www.abc.net.au/science/news/stories/s27924.htm

"Analyzing The Proliferation of Therapy"; CBS News; April 27, 2008; retrieved online on April 28, 2008 at http://www.cbsnews.com/stories/2008/04/27/sunday/main4048474.shtml.

BBC News; "Depression leads to worst health"; retrieved online on June 20, 2008 at http://news.bbc.co.uk/2/hi/health/6981678.stm.

BBC News; "Exercise to treat depression call"; March 28, 2005; retrieved online March 28, 2008 from http://news.bbc.co.uk/2/hi/health/4378389.stm.

Briley, John; "Working Out Your Issues"; *Washington Post*; June 14, 2005; retrieved online on June 16, 2008 at http://www.washingtonpost.com/wp-dyn/content/article/2005/06/13/AR2005061301418_pf.html.

Broussard-Wilson, Samantha; "Study finds link between exercise, mental health"; Yale Daily News; December 4, 2007; retrieved online January 11, 2008 at http://www.yaledailynews.com/articles/view/22691.

Cynkar, Amy; "A prescription for exercise"; *Monitor on Psychology* Volume 38, No. 6 June 2007; retrieved online on March 28, 2008 at http://www.apa.org/monitor/jun07/prescription.html.

Forliti, Amy; "Exercise Helps Treat Depression"; The Associated Press; March 17, 2005; retrieved online on December 28, 2007 at http://www.cbsnews.com/ stories/2005/03/17/health/ main681456.shtml.

Hamilton, Carey; "Critics question use of antidepressants"; *The Salt Lake Tribune*; September 5, 2003; purchased from the *Tribune* 's online archives on April 16, 2008.

Hawryluk, Markian; "Outrunning Depression"; *Bend* (OR) *Bulletin* ; 12/20/07; E1.

Helliker, Kevin; "How exercise can help fight depression"; *Wall Street Journal* ; May 10, 2005.

Johnson, Thomas; "Alternative Ways of Supporting Individuals Struggling With Depression"; International Center for Psychiatry and Psychology, Summer 2004 Newsletter.

Karp, Hannah; "Working Out Your Anxiety"; Wall Street Journal; August 11, 2006; retrieved online on June 20, 2008 at http://www.smartproinsight.com/ wallstreetjournal081106.htm.

Kolata, Gina; "Yes, Running Can Make You High"; *New York Times*; 3/27/08; retrieved online on 4/14/08 at http://www.nytimes.com/2008/03/27/health/ nutrition/27best.html

Langreth, Robert; "Patient Fix Thyself"; Forbes. com, April 9, 2007; retrieved online April 27, 2008 at http://www.forbes.com/forbes/2007/0409/080.html.

Marano, Hara Estroff; "Depression Lowers Productivity"; *Psychology Today* Jul/Aug 2003; retrieved online April 30, 2008 from http://psychologytoday.com/articles/pto-20030722-000001.html.

Rojas, Aurelio; "Assembly bill sweats the details"; 4/26/08; retrieved online on April 30, 2008 at http://www.sacbee.com/health/story/891720.html.

"Runners High Demonstrated: Brain Imaging Shows Release Of Endorphins In Brain"; *Science Daily*; retrieved online on April 14, 2008 at http://www.sciencedaily.com/releases/2008/03/080303101110.htm.

Schoen, Gwen; "Nutrition IQ"; *Sacramento Bee*; February 10, 2008; p. L8.

Yeung, Rob; "Racing to euphoria"; *New Scientist*; 11/23/96; retrieved online on 4/20/08 at http://www.newscientist.com/article/mg15220574.300-racing-to-euphoria.html.

General Reference

Baker, Jo-Anne; "Getting The Most Out Of Your Sex Life: Practitioner and Client Issues"; RedOrbit.com; posted November 30, 2007; retrieved online on April 4,

2008 at http://www.redorbit.com/news/health/1163572/getting_the_most_out_of_your_sex_life_practitioner_and/index.html.

"Can Exercise Make Me High?"; HealthCentral.com; retrieved December 28, 2007 at http://www.healthcentral.com/fitorfat/408/41285.html.

"Depression and anxiety: Exercise eases symptoms"; MayoClinic.com; retrieved on December 28, 2007 at http://www.mayoclinic.com/health/depression-and-exercise/MH00043.

"Depression & Anxiety: What To Do When Your Antidepressant Doesn't Work"; e-mail received 6/25/08 from Johns Hopkins Health Alerts (johnshopkins@johnshopkinshealthalerts.com).

"Exercise Helps Keep Your Psyche Fit"; American Psychological Association; May 28, 2004; retrieved online on December 28, 2007 at http://www.psychologymatters.org/exercise.html.

"Exercise for Depression: Background Research"; Depression Alliance Scotland; retrieved online on December 28, 2007 at http://www.dascot.org/exercise_research.html.

Hays, Kate F.; *Working It Out: Using Exercise in Psychotherapy*; American Psychological Association; Washington, D.C.; 1999.

Johnsgard, Keith; *Conquering Depression and Anxiety Through Exercise*; Prometheus Books; 2004.

Johnsgard, Keith, Ph.D.; *The Exercise Prescription for Depression and Anxiety*; Plenum Press; New York, NY; 1989.

Johnson, Thomas; "Alternative Ways of Supporting Individuals Struggling With Depression"; International Center for Psychiatry and Psychology, Summer 2004 Newsletter; retrieved online January 11, 2008 at http://www.icspp.org/index.php?option=com_content&task=view&id=17&Itemid=41.

Jones, Martin; "Promoting mental health through physical activity: examples form practice"; Journal of Mental Health Promotion March 2004; retrieved online on March 26, 2008 at http://www.findarticles.com/p/articles/mi_qa4122/is_200403/ai_n9465303.

"Just the expectation of a mirthful laughter experience boosts endorphins 27 percent, HGH 87 percent"; American Physiological Society press release; April 3, 2006; retrieved online on May 5, 2008 at http://www.eurekalert.org/pub_releases/2006-04/aps-jte033006.php.

Leith, Larry M.; *Exercising Your Way to Better Mental Health*; Fitness Information Technology, Inc.; Morgantown, WV; 1998.

"Master of the Mind; Teaneck Addiction Researcher Coined Term 'Endorphins'"; RedOrbit.com; September 14, 2004; retrieved online on March 20, 2008 at http://www.redorbit.com/news/science/86241/master_of_the_mind__teaneck_addiction_researcher_coined_term/

Mueller, Beth; "Massage leads to increased endorphin levels"; SpineHealth.com; May 10, 2002; retrieved online on April 4, 2008 at http://www.spine-health.com/Wellness/Massage-Therapy/About-Massage-Therapy/Massage-Therapy-For-Lower-Back-Pain.html.

Panning, Jennifer C.; "Mental Health Benefits of Exercise"; FindCounseling.com Mental Health Journal November 200; retrieved online on January 11, 2008 at http://www.findcounseling.com/journal/health-fitness/.

Ratey, John J. MD with Eric Hagerman; *Spark: The Revolutionary New Science of Exercise and the Brain*; Little, Brown and Company; New York, NY; 2008.

"SAMHSA Report Examines a Decade of Spending on Mental Health and Substance Abuse Treatment," *Psychiatr Serv* 56:767-768, June 2005; retrieved online April 3, 2008 from http://www.psychservices.psychiatryonline.org/cgi/content/full/56/6/767

"The Science of Chocolate"; BBC.co.uk; November 17, 2004; retrieved on April 4, 2008 from http://

www.bbc.co.uk/science/hottopics/chocolate/addictive.shtml.

U.S. Department of Health and Human Services; *The Effects of Physical Activity on Health and Disease: A Report of the Surgeon General*; 1996; p.135.

#

Endnotes

1   U.S. Department of Health and Human Services; *The Effects of Physical Activity on Health and Disease: A Report of the Surgeon General*; 1996; p.135.

2   It's important to note that while exercise has proven to be an effective remedy for some people, it won't necessarily work for everyone experiencing depression. "Depression" is a generic term that covers a wide range of experiences and symptoms. Diagnosed depression may be mild or moderate or severe, it may be situational or chronic, it may be the single issue present or just one aspect of a more complex condition such as bipolar disorder (a.k.a. manic depression). Some people's symptoms will respond to some forms of treatment and others inevitably will not. And most people suffering from depression will benefit from individual psychotherapy of some sort, whether it's traditional talk therapy or cognitive behavioral therapy.

3   U.S. Department of Health and Human Services; *The Effects of Physical Activity on Health and Disease: A Report of the Surgeon General*; 1996; p.135.

4   Langreth, Robert; "Patient Fix Thyself"; Forbes. com, April 9, 2007; retrieved online April 27, 2008

at http://www.forbes.com/forbes/2007/0409/080.html.

5   Jeff Greenfield; "Analyzing The Proliferation Of Therapy"; CBS News; 4/27/08; retrieved online on 4/28/08 from http://www.cbsnews.com/stories/2008/04/27/Sunday/main4048474.shtml

6   Carey Hamilton; "Critics question use of anti-depressants"; *The Salt Lake Tribune*; September 5, 2003; retrieved online April 16, 2008 from http://www.sltrib.com.

7   "Between 20 and 30 percent of depression patients don't respond to medication after a year of taking it, says Douglas G. Jacobs, associate clinical professor of psychiatry at Harvard Medical School." Kevin Helliker; "How exercise can help fight depression"; *Wall Street Journal* ; May 10, 2005.

8   G.E. Simon, M. VonKorff, W. Barlow; "Health care costs of primary care patients with recognized depression"; *Archives of General Psychiatry*, 52, 850-856. Cited in Wayne T. Philips, Ph.D., Michaela Kernan, Ph.D., Abby C. King, Ph.D.; "Physical Activity as a Nonpharmacological Treatment for Depression: A Review"; *Complementary Health Practice Review* Vol. 8 No. 2 April 2003; p. 139.

9   Hara Estroff Marano; "Depression Lowers Productivity"; *Psychology Today* Jul/Aug 2003; retrieved online April 30, 2008 from http://psychologytoday.com/articles/pto-20030722-000001.html.

10   Martin Jones; "Promoting mental health through physical activity: examples from practice"; *Journal of Mental Health Promotion*; March 2004.

11   Amanda J. Daley; "Exercise therapy and mental health in clinical populations: is exercise therapy a worthwhile intervention?"; *Advances in Psychiatric Treatment* (2002) 8: 262-270.

12   BBC News; "Exercise to treat depression call"; March 28, 2005; retrieved online March 28, 2008 from http://news.bbc.co.uk/2/hi/health/4378389.stm.

13   "In era of pills, fewer shrinks doing talk therapy"; The Associated Press; August 4, 2008; retrieved online on August 4, 2008 at http://www.msnbc.msn.com/id/26011514/.

14   W.P. Morgan; "A pilot investigation of physical working capacity in depressed and nondepressed psychiatric males"; *Research Quarterly* (1969), 4:859-861. Cited in E.W. Martinsen; "Exercise and Depression"; *International Journal of Sport and Exercise Psychology* (2005) 3(4):469-483.

15   Martinsen; "Exercise and Depression"; 471.

16   S.L. Franz & G.V. Hamilton; "Effects of exercise upon the retardation in condition of depression"; *American Journal of Insanity* (1905), 62:239-256. Cited in Martinsen; "Exercise and Depression"; 472.

17   Griest, J.H., Klein, M.H., Eischens, R.R., Gurman, A.S. & Morgan, W.P. "Running as treatment for depression"; *Comprehensive Psychiatry* (1979), 20:41-54. Cited in Martinsen; "Exercise and Depression"; 472.

18   Klein, M.H., Griest, J.H., Gurman, A.S., Neimeyer, R.A., Lesser, D.P., Bushnell, N.J. & Smith, R.E. "A comparative outcome study of group psychother-apy vs. exercise treatments for depression"; *International Journal of Mental Health* (1985), 13:148-177. Cited in Martinsen; "Exercise and Depression"; 472.

19   For example, the studies led by James A. Blumen-thal and Michael Babyak of Duke University, and by Andrea L. Dunn of the Cooper Institute and Madhukat H. Trivedi of the University of Texas. See A.L. Dunn, M.H. Trivedi, J.B. Kampert, C.G. Clark, H.O. Chambliss; "Exercise Treatment for Depression"; American Journal of Preventative Medicine (2005) 28:1; and J.A. Blumenthal, M.A. Babyak, K.A. Moore, W.A. Craighead, S. Her-man, P. Khatri, R. Waugh, M.A. Napolitano, P.M. Doraiswami, K.R. Krishnan; "Effects of exercise training on older adults with major depression"; *Archives of Internal Medicine* (199), 159:2349-56.

20   For example: T. Christian North, Penny Mc-Cullagh & Zung Vu Tran; "Effect of Exercise on Depression"; *Exercise and Sport Science Reviews* (1989), 18:379-415; and Daley; "Exercise therapy and mental health in clinical populations: is exer-cise therapy a worthwhile intervention?" 262-270. The quote is from Gregg A. Tkachuk and Garry L. Martin; "Exercise Therapy for Patients With Psy-chiatric Disorders: Research and Clinical Implica-tions"; *Professional Psychology: Research and Practice* (1999), 30(3):275-282.

21   Martinsen; "Exercise and Depression"; 472. More recently, researchers have used positron emission tomography to confirm that cognitive behavioral therapy causes lasting physiological changes in brain function comparable to antidepressant medication—but without the side effects (Langreth; "Patient Fix Thyself"; 4).

22   Michael Babyak, James A. Blumenthal, Steve Herman, Parinda Khatri, Murali Doraiswamy, Kathleen Moore, Edward Craighead, Teri T. Baldewicz, K. Ranga Krishnan; "Exercise Treatment for Major Depression: Maintenance of Therapeutic Benefit at 10 Months"; Psychosomatic Medicine 62:633-638 (2000). In a twist the researchers called "unexpected," patients in the group that both exercised and received medication received no more benefit than the groups that received only one or the other treatment. In fact, "several in the combined group mentioned spontaneously that the medication seemed to interfere with the beneficial effects of the exercise program."

23   Wayne T. Phillips, Michaela Kiernan, Abby C. King; "Physical Activity as a Nonpharmacological Treatment for Depression: A Review"; Complementary Health Practice Review (2003) 8:139-152; p.144.

24   Lynette L. Craft; "Exercise and clinical depression: examining two psychological mechanisms"; Psychology of Sport and Exercise (2005) 6(2):151-171.

25   Ibid.

26   Tkachuk and Martin; "Exercise Therapy for Patients With Psychiatric Disorders: Research and

Clinical Implications"; 276. Tkachuk and Martin cite two studies as sources for this finding: Freemont, J., & Craighead, L. W.; "Aerobic exercise and cognitive therapy in the treatment of dysphoric moods"; *Cognitive Therapy and Research* (1987), 11:241-251; and Greist et al; "Running as a treatment for depression."

27   North, McCullagh & Tran, "Effect of Exercise on Depression"; 403.

28   Ibid, 406.

29   Ibid, 406.

30   J.A. Horne & C.H. Staff; "Exercise and sleep: Body heating effects"; *Sleep* (1983) 6:36-46; referenced in Daley; "Exercise therapy and mental health in clinical populations: is exercise therapy a worthwhile intervention?"

31   Martinsen; "Exercise and Depression"; 474.

32   North, McCullagh & Tran; "Effect of Exercise on Depression"; 407.

33   "Master of the Mind; Teaneck Addiction Researcher Coined Term 'Endorphins'"; RedOrbit. com; September 14, 2004; retrieved online on March 20, 2008 at http://www.redorbit.com/news/science/86241/master_of_the_mind__teaneck_addiction_researcher_coined_term/.

34   North, McCullagh & Tran; "Effect of Exercise on Depression"; 407, citing C.B. Pert & D.L. Bowie; "Behavioral manipulation of rats causes alterations in opiate receptor occupancy"; in E. Usdin, W.E. Bunney & N.S. Kline (eds.); *Endorphins in Mental*

Health; New York, Oxford University Press, 1979, 93-104.

35   Daley; "Exercise therapy and mental health in clinical populations: is exercise therapy a worthwhile intervention?"; 265-266.

36   Michael Artal with Carl Sherman; "Exercise Against Depression"; *The Physician and Sportsmedicine* (1998), 26(10); retrieved online April 3, 2008 at http://www.physsportsmed.com/issues/1998/10Oct/artal.htm.

37   Rob Yeung; "Racing to euphoria"; *New Scientist*; 11/23/96; retrieved online on 4/20/08 at http://www.newscientist.com/article/mg15220574.300-racing-to-euphoria.html.

38   For example, Kevin Helliker's *Wall Street Journal* piece and Markian Hawryluk; "Outrunning Depression"; *Bend* (OR) *Bulletin* ; 12/20/07; E1.

39   Martinsen; "Exercise and Depression"; 475.

40   "The myth of runner's high revisited with brain imaging"; University of Bonn news release; 3/3/08; retrieved online on 4/14/08 at http://www.eurekalert.org/pub/releases/2008-03/uob-tmo030308.php.

41   Ibid.

42   Ibid.

43   Gina Kolata; "Yes, Running Can Make You High"; *New York Times*; 3/27/08; retrieved online on 4/14/08 at http://www.nytimes.com/2008/03/27/health/nutrition/27best.html

44   Ibid.

45   "The Science of Chocolate"; BBC.co.uk; November 17, 2004; retrieved online on April 4, 2008 from http://www.bbc.co.uk/science/hottopics/chocolate/addictive.shtml.

46   While it is true that in the case of each alternative activity cited in this chapter, endorphin activity was measured via blood draws rather than PET scans, the Boecker experiment suggests a stronger correlation between endorphins in the bloodstream and endorphins inside the brain than has been previously established. As a result, we would anticipate that new endorphin research will follow Boecker et al's example and use PET scans to confirm that endorphins in the blood stream do correlate with endorphins in the brain to some as-yet-undefined degree.

47   Beth Mueller; "Massage leads to increased endorphin levels"; SpineHealth.com; May 10, 2002; retrieved online on April 4, 2008 at http://www.spine-health.com/Wellness/Massage-Therapy/About-Massage-Therapy/Massage-Therapy-For-Lower-Back-Pain.html.

48   "It seems inserting the fine needles into the specially-defined body points triggers the production of chemicals called endorphins."—C. Johnson; "Acupuncture works on endorphins"; News In Science, ABC.net; retrieved online on April 22, 2008 at: http://www.abc.net.au/science/news/stories/s27924.htm

49   American Physiological Society press release; "Just the expectation of a mirthful laughter ex-

perience boosts endorphins 27 percent, HGH 87 percent"; 4/3/06. The experiment cited was conducted by Lee S. Berk of Loma Linda University.

50   "Recent studies by Dr Candace Pert at Johns Hopkins University, USA, have documented that the production of endorphins increases 200% from sexual activity." Jo-Anne Baker; "Getting The Most Out Of Your Sex Life: Practitioner and Client Issues"; RedOrbit.com; Posted on: Friday, 30 November 2007.

51   John J. Ratey, MD with Eric Hagerman; *Spark: The Revolutionary New Science of Exercise and the Brain*; Little, Brown and Company; 2008; p.7.

52   Artal & Sherman; "Exercise Against Depression"; 4.

53   Dunn, Trivedi et al; "Exercise Treatment for Depression"; 7.

54   Mayo Clinic Staff; "Depression and Anxiety: Exercise eases symptoms"; retrieved online on December 28, 2007 at http://www/mayoclinic.com/health/depression-and-exercise/MH00043.

55   Helliker; "How exercise can help fight depression."

56   Pigott, H.E.; Leventhal, A.M. ; Alter, G.S.; Boren, J.J.; "Efficacy and Effectiveness of Antidepressants: Current Status of Research"; *Psychother Psychosom* 2010;79:267-279 (DOI:10.1159/000318293).

57   Elder, G.A.; De Gasperi, R.; Gama Sosa, M.A.; "Research update: neurogenesis in adult brain and neuropsychiatric disorders."; *Mt Sinai J Med.* 2006

Nov;73(7):931-40; Department of Psychiatry, Mount Sinai School of Medicine, New York, NY. Also: Jeremy Coplan, MD; "Update on Neurogenesis Research and Implications for Psychiatric Disorders—February 11, 2006"; retrieved online at http://neuroscienceupdate.cumc.columbia.edu/popups/transcript_coplan.html on September 3, 2010.

58   Jeffrey Schwartz and Sharon Begley; *The Mind and the Brain: Neuroplasticity and the Power of Mental Force*; Harper; 2002. Also: Sharon Begley; *Train Your Mind, Change Your Brain: How a New Science Reveals Our Extraordinary Potential to Transform Ourselves*; Ballantine; 2007.

59   Zindel V. Segal, PhD; J. Mark G. Williams, DPhil; and John D. Teasdale, PhD; *Mindfulness-Based Cognitive Therapy for Depression: A New Approach to Preventing Relapse*; The Guilford Press; 2002.

60   R.A. Emmons & M.E. McCullough; Journal of Personality and Social Psychology, 2003, 84, 377-89. Also: RA Emmons, PhD.; *Thanks! How the New Science of Gratitude Can Make You Happier*; Houghton Mifflin Company; 2007; and R.A. Emmons & M.E. McCullough, Editors; *The Psychology of Gratitude*; Oxford University Press; 2004.

61   Fred Luskin, PhD ; *Forgive for Good: A Proven Prescription for Health and Happiness*; HarperOne; 2003. Also Jack Kornfield; *The Art of Forgiveness, Lovingkindness, and Peace*; Bantam; 2008.

62   Martin L. Rossman, M.D.; *Guided Imagery for Self-Healing*; HJ Kramer/New World Library; 2000.

63   Gortner, E.M.; Rude, S.S.; Pennebaker, J.W.; "Benefits of expressive writing in lowering rumination and depressive symptoms."; *Behav Ther.* 2006 Sep;37(3):292-303; University of Texas at Austin.

64   James W. Pennebaker; *Writing to Heal: A guided journal for recovering from trauma & emotional upheaval*; New Harbinger Publications, Inc; 2004.

65   Barton, J; Pretty, J.; "What is the best dose of nature and green exercise for improving mental health? A multi-study analysis." *Environ Sci Technol.* 2010 May 15;44(10):3947-55. Interdisciplinary Centre for Environment and Society, Department of Biological Sciences, University of Essex, Colchester, U.K.

66   Neckelmann, D.; Mykletun, A.; Dahl, A.A.; "Chronic insomnia as a risk factor for developing anxiety and depression"; *Sleep* 2007 Jul 1;30(7):873-80; Department of Psychiatry, Clinic of Psychosomatic Medicine, Haukeland University Hospital, Bergen, Norway.

67   Walsh, F.; "Human-animal bonds I: the relational significance of companion animals."; *Fam Process* 2009 Dec; 48(4):462-80;Center for Family Health, University of Chicago.

68   Hirsch, R.D.; Junglas, K.; Konradt, B.; Jonitz, M.F.; "Humor therapy in the depressed elderly: results of an empirical study" [article in German]; *Z Gerontol Geriatr.* 2010 Feb;43(1):42-52.

69   Wen-Hsuan Hou; Pai-Tsung Chiang, Tun-Yen; Hsu, Su-Ying Chiu; Yung-Chieh Yen; "Treatment effects of massage therapy in depressed people: a meta-analysis."; *J Clin Psychiatry* 71(7):894-901 (2010); Department of Physical Medicine and Rehabilitation, Kaohsiung, Taiwan.

70   Gunter Kreutz, Stephan Bongard, Sonja Rohrmann, Volker Hodapp, Dorothee Grebe; "Effects of Choir Singing or Listening on Secretory Immunoglobulin A, Cortisol, and Emotional State"; 2003. Also: Bryan C. Hunter, PhD; "Singing as a Therapeutic Agent, in The Etude"; *Journal of Music Therapy*: Vol. 36, No. 2, pp. 125–143; Nazareth College, Rochester, New York, NY.

71   Dowlati, Y.; Herrmann, N.; Swardfager, W.; Liu, H.; Sham, L.; Reim, E.K.; Lanctôt, K.L.; "A meta-analysis of cytokines in major depression."; *Biol Psychiatry*, 2010 Mar 1;67(5):446-57; Department of Pharmacology and Toxicology, University of Toronto, Toronto, Ontario, Canada. Also: Beezhold, B.L.; Johnston, C.S.; Daigle, D.R.; "Vegetarian diets are associated with healthy mood states: a cross-sectional study in seventh day adventist adults."; *Nutr J.* 2010 Jun 1;9:26.; Department of Nutrition, Arizona State University, Mesa, Arizona.

72   Maes, M.; Christophe, A.; Delanghe, J.; Altamura, C.; Neels, H.; Meltzer, H.Y. "Lowered omega3 polyunsaturated fatty acids in serum phospholipids and cholesteryl esters of depressed patients."; *Psychiatry Res.* 1999;85:275-291.

73   Nemets, B.; Stahl, Z.; Belmaker, R.H. "Addition of omega-3 fatty acid to maintenance medication treatment for recurrent unipolar depressive disorder." *Am J Psychiatry.* 2002;159:477-479.

74   Su, K.P.; Huang, S.Y.; Chiu, C.C.; Shen, W.W. "Omega-3 fatty acids in major depressive disorder. A preliminary double-blind, placebo-controlled trial." *Eur Neuropsychopharmacol.* 2003;13:267-271.

75   Coppen, A.; Bolander-Gouaille, C.; "Treatment of depression: time to consider folic acid and vitamin B12."; *J Psychopharmacol.* 2005 Jan;19(1):59-65. MRC Neuropsychiatric Research Laboratory, Epsom, Surrey, UK.

76   Coppen, A.; Bailey, J.; "Enhancement of the antidepressant action of fluoxetine by folic acid: a randomised, placebo controlled trial." *J Affect Dis* 2000;60:121-31. Also: Kimberly A Skarupski, Christine Tangney, Hong Li, Bichun Ouyang, Denis A Evans, Martha Clare Morris; "Longitudinal association of vitamin B-6, folate, and vitamin B-12 with depressive symptoms among older adults over time"; *Am J Clin Nutr* (June 2, 2010).

77   Wilkins, C.H.; Sheline, Y.I.; Roe, C.M.; Birge, S.J.; Morris, J.C.; "Vitamin D deficiency is associated with low mood and worse cognitive performance in older adults."; *Am J Geriatr Psychiatry.* 2006 Dec;14(12):1032-40.

78   Buell, J.S.; Scott, T.M.; Dawson-Hughes, B.; Dallal, G.E.; Rosenberg, I.H.; Folstein, M.F.; Tucker, K.L.; "Vitamin D is associated with cognitive function in elders receiving home health services."; *J Gerontol A Biol Sci Med Sci.* 2009 Aug;64(8):888-95. Epub 2009 Apr 17.Jean Mayer USDA Human Nutrition Research Center on Aging, Tufts University, Boston, MA

79   Linde K, Ramirez G, Mulrow CD, et al.; "St. John's wort for depression: an overview and meta-analysis of randomized clinical trials."; *BMJ* 1996;313:253-8. Also: Gaster, B.; Holroyd, J. "St John's wort for depression."; *Arch Intern Med* 2000;160:152-6.

80   Bressa, G.M.; "S-adenosyl-l-methionine (SAMe) as antidepressant: meta-analysis of clinical studies." *Acta Neurol Scand Suppl* 1994;154:7-14.

81   Shaw, K.; Turner, J.; Del Mar, C.; "Tryptophan and 5-hydroxytryptophan for depression." *Cochrane Database Syst Rev* 2002;(1):CD003198.

82   Levine, J.; Barak, Y.; Gonzalves, M,; et al. "Double-blind, controlled trial of inositol treatment of depression." *Am J Psychiatry* 1995;152:792-4.

83   Logan, A.; Katzman, M.; "Major depressive disorder: probiotics may be an adjuvant therapy." *Med Hypotheses* 2005;64:533–8. Also: Benton, D.; Williams, C.; Brown, A.; "Impact of consuming a milk drink containing a probiotic on mood and cognition."; *Eur J Clin Nutr.* 2007;61:355–61. Also: A. Venket Rao, Alison C. Bested, Tracey M. Beaulne, Martin A. Katzman, Christina Iorio,

John M. Berardi, Alan C. Logan; "A randomized, double-blind, placebo-controlled pilot study of a probiotic in emotional symptoms of chronic fatigue syndrome"; *Gut Pathog.* 2009; 1: 6.; published online 2009 March 19.

84   Daley; "Exercise therapy and mental health in clinical populations: is exercise therapy a worthwhile intervention?"; p. 267.

85   W.E. Sime; "Guidelines for clinical applications of exercise therapy for mental health" in J.L. Van Raalte & B.W. Brwer (Eds.); *Exploring sport and exercise psychology* (pp. 159-187); Washington, D.C. American Psychological Association. Cited in Tkachuk & Martin; "Exercise Therapy for Patients With Psychiatric Disorders: Research and Clinical Implications," 280.

86   John Briley; "Working Out Your Issues"; *The Washington Post*; June 14, 2005; retrieved online on June 17, 2008 at http://www.washington-post.com/wp-dyn/content/article/2005/06/13/AR2005061301418_pf.html.

87   "In era of pills, fewer shrinks doing talk therapy"; The Associated Press; August 4, 2008; retrieved online on August 4, 2008 at http://www.msnbc.msn.com/id/26011514/.

88   Markian Hawryluk; "Outrunning depression"; *Bend Bulletin*; 12/20/07; the article lead appears on page E1 and quote is from the jump on E8.

89   Hawryluk; "Outrunning depression"; E8.

90   U.S. Department of Health and Human Services; *The Effects of Physical Activity on Health and Disease: A Report of the Surgeon General*; 1996; p. 150.

91   Hawryluk; "Outrunning Depression"; E1.

92   "Exercise Helps Keep Your Psyche Fit"; retrieved online on June 20, 2008 at http://www.psychologymatters.org/exercise.html.

93   Notably, Keith Helliker's "How exercise can fight depression" appeared in May 2005 followed by Hannah Karp's "Working out your anxiety" in August 2006.

94   "Let's Talk Facts About Depression"; American Psychiatric Association; 2005; retrieved online on June 20, 2008 at http://www.healthyminds.org/multimedia/depression.pdf.

95   Ratey; *Spark: The Revolutionary New Science of Exercise and the Brain*; p. 126. Dr. Ratey's observations were of course made prior to the publication of the Boecker endorphin study.

96   "Depression & Anxiety: What To Do When Your Antidepressant Doesn't Work"; e-mail received 6/25/08 from Johns Hopkins Health Alerts (johnshopkins@johnshopkinshealthalerts.com).

97   Helliker; "How exercise can fight depression."

98   "Exercise to treat depression call"; BBC News; 3/28/05; retrieved online on 12/28/07 at http://news.bbc.co.uk/1/hi/health/4378389.stm.

99   BBC News; "Depression leads to worst health"; retrieved online on June 20, 2008 at http://news.bbc.co.uk/2/hi/health/6981678.stm.

100   Aurelio Rojas; "Assembly bill sweats the details"; 4/26/08; retrieved online on April 30, 2008 at http://www.sacbee.com/health/story/891720.html.